Safe Sedation for All Practitioners
A Practical Guide

Safe Sedation for All Practitioners
A Practical Guide

JAMES WATTS BSc MB ChB FRCA
Consultant in Anaesthesia and Intensive Care Medicine
East Lancashire Hospitals Trust

Radcliffe Publishing
Oxford • New York

Radcliffe Publishing Ltd
18 Marcham Road
Abingdon
Oxon OX14 1AA
United Kingdom

www.radcliffe-oxford.com
Electronic catalogue and worldwide online ordering facility.

British Library Cataloguing in Publication Data

A catalogue record for this book is available from the British Library.

ISBN-13: 978 184619 220 3

Typeset by Pindar New Zealand, (Egan Reid), Auckland, New Zealand
Printed and bound by TJ International Ltd, Padstow, Cornwall, UK

Contents

Preface

Sedative adj. having a calming effect. *n.* a sedative drug.

The Oxford Popular English Dictionary (2001)

Anaesthesia is one of the Victorians' most important legacies for the modern world. Prior to its introduction, surgery was by necessity brutal and fast, as methods of pain relief were only partially effective at best. The ability to perform painless surgery has been regarded as one of the greatest human achievements, and the development of anaesthesia has been recognised by both the public and the medical profession as one of the top three medical milestones of the last 170 years.[1] However, there are a great many procedures and treatments for which full general anaesthesia is regarded as too great an intervention, but for which a state of reduced anxiety and consciousness is still necessary. This state is referred to as 'sedation.' The term is used ubiquitously in many contexts in the healthcare setting, but this text will be confined to a discussion of sedation as a means of allowing patients to comfortably undergo some form of medical intervention, or of circumstances in which sedation is used as a defined part of a medical treatment.

It is relevant to ask why a book on the basics of sedation practice is required if sedation is already widely used throughout the healthcare sector. However, it should be appreciated that sedating a patient is not a risk-free enterprise. There is an assumption that the act of sedation is inherently safer than inducing general anaesthesia, although there is no real evidence base to support this belief. Some authorities have suggested that there is a 1 in 2000 risk of 30-day mortality associated with the use of sedation (usually due to cardiovascular or respiratory problems), compared with an estimated mortality of around 1 in 100 000 for general anaesthesia. Other analyses have shown that 14% of patients undergoing endoscopy received a sedative overdose. In addition, medical procedures themselves can be associated with physiological problems such as hypoxia or cardiac abnormalities – phenomena which sedation itself might exacerbate.[2-4]

If there are serious problems with regard to the way that sedation is performed, one could ask why guidelines have not been formulated to standardise practice. In fact many guidelines exist, but there is evidence that they are not universally adhered to. The reasons for this are legion. Some groups of practitioners may consider that certain guidelines do not apply to their field of practice, while others may feel that, due to a lack of proper randomised controlled trials, the guidelines are not evidence based and are therefore open to challenge. Furthermore, there is a lack of formal training in sedative techniques in non-anaesthetic medical specialties, and so there is good reason to believe that knowledge with regard to basic safe practices, as well as ignorance of existing guidelines, may be a problem. Finally, many non-medically and non-dentally trained healthcare practitioners, who may not necessarily have access to the guidelines produced by a specialist association, are providing sedation for an increasing variety of interventions. It is clearly essential for everyone in the team that is caring for the patient to have the same understanding of the principles and issues involved. Therefore the question inevitably arises as to why, if the situation is so fraught with hazards, the administration of sedation is not restricted solely to those with anaesthetic training. The answer, of course, is that demand for sedation greatly outstrips the supply of anaesthetists. However, there is a good argument for believing that anaesthetists should be heavily involved in the quality control of non-anaesthetic sedation services, even if they themselves cannot actively participate.

Sedation is a tool that requires care if it is to be used correctly. The modern sedationist must therefore be able to demonstrate that they can practise safely. This means that they should be able to produce evidence that they have undergone adequate training in relevant skills, and that they have maintained and developed those skills. This requires a sound understanding of the basic sciences involved, and an intimate knowledge of the standards of practice that should be adhered to. The aim of this book is to be useful in this regard to any sedationist from any background. It is intended to be a first-line educational resource for those who are training in the techniques of sedation, and also for those who already practise, but who wish to consolidate their knowledge in a structured way. It is hoped that it will provide a rational syllabus that is easy to use, and that will provide sedationists at any level of experience with a firm basis on which to develop their practice, grounded upon a sound understanding of basic principles, including patient selection and assessment, pharmacology, monitoring equipment and legal issues. These precepts are illustrated throughout by relevant clinical scenarios derived from real-life situations. Where appropriate, these have been attributed to the relevant sources. Where the scenarios are unattributed, they are derived from personal communications with fellow clinicians who wish to remain anonymous.

What this book does *not* aim to do is to provide a 'one method fits every situation' recipe for sedation. The experienced and safe sedationist should, of course, be able to adapt their practice appropriately depending upon circumstances and, most importantly, to recognise when they have reached the limits of their competency and more expert assistance is required.

James Watts
January 2008

References

1 Medical milestones. Celebrating key advances since 1840. *BMJ.* 2007; **334 (Supplement).**

2 Quine MA, Bell GD, McCloy RF *et al.* A prospective audit of upper gastrointestinal endoscopy in two regions of England: safety, staffing and sedation methods. *Gut.* 1995; **36:** 462–7.

3 Jenkins K, Baker AB. Consent and anaesthetic risk. *Anaesthesia.* 2003; **58:** 962–84.

4 National Confidential Enquiry into Patient Outcome and Death. *Scoping Our Practice*; www.ncepod.org.uk/pdf/2004/04sum.pdf (accessed 27 June 2007).

About the author

James Watts graduated from the University of St Andrews in 1986 and the University of Manchester in 1989. He has been a Consultant in Anaesthesia and Intensive Care Medicine in the North West of England since 1998, during which time he has held the posts of Clinical Director, Deputy Medical Director and Joint Lead Clinician for the Lancashire and South Cumbria Critical Care Network, to name but a few. He has led his clinical team into the finals of the 2002 British Association of Medical Managers (BAMM) Medical Management Team of the Year and the 2006 Hospital Doctor Awards.

For Jennifer and the boys.
Jih-oh!

CHAPTER 1

Sedation for procedures, treatments and investigations: a general introduction

Terms to be used

It is important that the proper meanings of terms used throughout this book are clearly understood, in order to avoid confusion. For this reason, terminology that is used frequently in the text is listed in Table 1.1 below.

TABLE 1.1 Definition of terms commonly used within this book

TERM	DEFINITION
AAGBI	The Association of Anaesthetists of Great Britain and Ireland.
Airway	The anatomical area from the nasal passages to the alveoli in the lungs, consisting of the nasopharynx, the oropharynx, the larynx, the trachea, the bronchi, the bronchioles and the alveoli. A *patent airway* is one that is not occluded in any way.
Anaesthesia	A state characterised by a loss of sensation and depressed consciousness, resulting in a total lack of response to a painful procedure, such as a surgical incision.
Anaesthetic	A drug that is usually administered with the intention of inducing an anaesthetised state.
Anaesthetist	A practitioner who has been specifically trained to administer anaesthesia. In the UK, this is currently exclusively a doctor.
Analgesia	A reduction in the sensation of pain.

cont.

TERM	DEFINITION
Analgesic	A drug administered with the main aim of reducing pain.
Anxiolysis	A reduction in anxiety. This may be achieved by non-pharmacological means, but when induced by the administration of drugs this equates to a state defined as 'minimal sedation' (*see* Table 1.3).
Anxiolytic	A drug administered with the main aim of inducing anxiolysis.
Drug	A pharmacologically active chemical that has an effect upon a patient's physiology. A drug will usually (but not always) exert its effect when it reaches the *active site* of a *specific receptor*.
GDC	The General Dental Council, the regulatory body of the dental profession.
GMC	The General Medical Council, the regulatory body of the medical profession.
Hypercarbia	Raised carbon dioxide levels in a patient's blood or lungs.
Hypoxia	Reduced oxygen levels in a patient's blood or lungs.
Muscle relaxant	A drug administered with the specific aim of inducing muscle paralysis during anaesthesia. Also known as a neuromuscular blocker or a 'paralysing agent.'
NMC	The Nursing and Midwifery Council, the regulatory body of the nursing and midwifery professions.
Observer	Any individual who is monitoring a patient's condition.
Operator	Any person who is performing a medical procedure or investigation.
Operator-sedationist	Any person who is performing a medical procedure or investigation and who is also providing or supervising the sedation of the patient.
Paralysis	Relaxation of the muscles caused by the administration of a muscle relaxant (neuromuscular blocker).
RCoA	The Royal College of Anaesthetists.
Sedation	The administration of a drug or drugs in order to allow performance of a medical procedure or investigation. Verbal contact with the patient is maintained (see more detailed discussion of definitions below).
Sedationist	Any practitioner who is administering sedation to a patient.
Sedative drug	Any drug that is administered to a patient with the main aim of inducing a sedative effect.
Surgeon	Any practitioner who has been specifically trained to perform surgery.
Ventilation	Artificial ventilation of a patient's lungs by means of a mechanical or hand-powered ventilatory device, in order to prevent hypoxia.

Definition of sedation

The first principle of safe practice is to know exactly what is meant by the term 'sedation', and thereby to gain a firm understanding of what can, and cannot, be achieved when it is utilised. The word 'sedation' is commonly used as a generic term, implying the 'calming' of a patient.

A simple general description of sedation for the purpose of medical procedures would be as follows:

> A technique in which a drug or drugs produce depression of the central nervous system, enabling treatment to be carried out without physical or psychological stress, but during which verbal contact with the patient is maintained.

This definition is compiled from those used in many reports published by a variety of professional bodies. Some of the reports include the qualification that:

> The drug(s) and techniques used should have a wide margin of safety that makes accidental loss of consciousness unlikely.

A selection of the relevant guidelines is shown in Table 1.2.

TABLE 1.2 Selection of relevant professional guidelines on sedation

AUTHOR	REFERENCE
Standing Dental Advisory Committee	*General Anaesthesia, Sedation and Resuscitation in Dentistry. Report of an Expert Working Party (The Poswillo Report)*. London: Department of Health; 1990.
Joint Working Party of the Royal College of Radiologists and the Royal College of Anaesthetists	*Sedation and Anaesthesia in Radiology: Recommendations of the Joint Working Party of the Royal College of Radiologists and the Royal College of Anaesthetists*. London: Royal College of Anaesthetists; 1992.
Joint Working Party on Anaesthesia in Ophthalmic Surgery	*Report of the Joint Working Party on Anaesthesia in Ophthalmic Surgery*. London: Association of Anaesthetists of Great Britain and Ireland and the Royal College of Ophthalmologists; 1993.
Working Party on Guidelines for Sedation by the Non-Anaesthetist	*Report of the Working Party on Guidelines for Sedation by the Non-Anaesthetist*. London: Royal College of Surgeons of England; 1993.
American Society of Anesthesiologists	*Continuum of Depth of Sedation. Definition of General Anesthesia and Levels of Sedation/Analgesia*. Park Ridge, IL: American Society of Anesthesiologists; 1999.

cont.

AUTHOR	REFERENCE
American Academy of Pediatrics and American Academy of Pediatric Dentistry	*Guidelines for the Monitoring and Management of Pediatric Patients During and After Sedation for Diagnostic and Therapeutic Procedures: an update.* Elk Grove Village, IL: American Academy of Pediatrics; 2006.

This definition of sedation is seemingly straightforward, but the implication is that sedation is not a well-defined 'end point', but rather a continuum between the fully awake and the fully anaesthetised state.[1-3]

More precise definitions of the different possible levels of sedation have been suggested, and are listed in Table 1.3. These terms will be used again during the course of this book. It is obvious from reading these definitions that the transition between one level and another is quite 'soft', and that as a result it may be difficult to isolate chronologically when the patient becomes 'deeply sedated.' The transition to a level of *general anaesthesia* is, by contrast, very clear, because the patient becomes unresponsive to normal stimuli.

It therefore follows that whoever is administering the sedation to the patient must ensure that the patient's well-being is adequately monitored, and must be prepared to deal with the consequences of unanticipated problems, including the attainment of a deeper level of sedation than was intended. *In addition, it should be noted that, in the UK, deep sedation/analgesia is regarded as part of the spectrum of general anaesthesia, and not as a 'level of sedation.' Therefore the management of deep sedation in the UK is assumed to require training to the same standards of vigilance and skill as those required by an anaesthetist.*[4] The term 'deep sedation' can therefore be equated to a state of 'light anaesthesia', although many anaesthetists would dispute that such a state exists (i.e. a patient is either anaesthetised, or they are not). This also means that studies of sedation practice from the USA and the UK may differ greatly in what they are attempting to achieve, and so the resulting recommendations may also not be universally applicable.

It can be concluded from this that a sedative drug is a medication that globally depresses the functions of the central nervous system (CNS). Although this will have the advantage of reducing anxiety and inducing calm, it can also lead to loss of protective airway reflexes, and depression of respiratory and cardiovascular systems. It has been estimated that in paediatric sedation, the incidence of significant hypoxia may be 0.4%.[5]

The notion that sedation is a drug-induced interim state somewhere between full consciousness and anaesthesia, and that it is a continuum rather than a single well-defined entity, can be a difficult one for a training sedationist to grasp. In order to consolidate understanding of what sedation actually is, it is therefore also helpful to define exactly what it is *not*. Sedation is *not* synonymous with the terms 'analgesia' or 'muscle relaxation.' For example, sedation will help a patient to remain calm and relaxed for a bronchoscopy examination, but will not abolish the discomfort of a bronchoscope passing through the nasal passages or larynx; it will help a patient to remain comfortable on an operating table, but will not stop them reacting to a surgeon's incision.

TABLE 1.3 Definitions of the levels of sedation

LEVEL	DEFINITION
Minimal sedation (anxiolysis)	A drug-induced state during which the patient responds normally to verbal commands. Although cognitive function and coordination may be impaired, ventilatory and cardiovascular functions are unaffected.
Moderate sedation/ analgesia (conscious sedation/relative analgesia)	A drug-induced depression of consciousness, during which the patient responds purposefully to verbal commands, either alone or accompanied by light tactile stimulation (reflex withdrawal from a painful stimulus is not a purposeful response). No interventions are required to maintain a patent airway, and spontaneous ventilation is adequate. Cardiovascular function is usually maintained.
Deep sedation/ analgesia	A drug-induced depression of consciousness during which the patient cannot easily be roused but does respond purposefully following repeated or painful stimulation. The ability to maintain ventilatory function may be impaired. The patient may require assistance in maintaining a patent airway, and spontaneous ventilation may be inadequate. Cardiovascular function is usually maintained.
General anaesthesia	A drug-induced loss of consciousness during which the patient is not rousable even by painful stimulation. The ability to independently maintain ventilatory function is often impaired. Patients often require assistance in maintaining a patent airway, and positive pressure ventilation may be necessary because of depressed spontaneous ventilation or drug-induced depression of neuromuscular function. Cardiovascular function may be impaired.

Analgesia

Analgesia has a very specific meaning, namely a reduction in the sensation of pain. This concept is very easily understood, because pain is either present or it is not – and if it is present, a therapeutic intervention may reduce the sensation completely, partially or not at all.

Many different medications can be used to reduce the sensation of pain.

They can either be administered to or near the site of pain (such as a local anaesthetic injection), or they can be administered systemically to the whole patient (by inhalation, ingestion, injection, etc.). Some of these drugs have very powerful side-effects, which *may* include sedation. However, sedation is not the main effect of the drug, and so the fact that it has sedative side-effects does not mean that the drug can safely be used with the intention of inducing a sedative state. Sedative effects may in fact make the drug hazardous to use in some circumstances, or difficult to use in combination with actual sedatives, as the effects may be additive and unpredictable.

In contrast, most sedative drugs do not have a pain-relieving effect. Therefore the induction of a sedative state will *not* be expected to reduce the sensation of pain.

Muscle relaxation

Within anaesthesia, this is a term that has a very specific definition, namely the administration of neuromuscular blocking agents to a patient in order to relax (i.e. totally paralyse) the muscles in order to allow surgery or positive pressure ventilation. These drugs will all stop the patient breathing for a significant period of time, and require that ventilation is actively supported to prevent the patient from dying of hypoxia. The use of such muscle relaxants will render the patient totally immobile, which may mask any signs that the patient is actually fully awake rather than anaesthetised.

Muscle-paralysing agents should *not* be used as part of any sedative regime, nor should they even be drawn up into a syringe unless a person specifically trained in their use is present.

Outside of anaesthesia, the term 'muscle relaxation' can refer to the effect of drugs that reduce muscle tension. Some sedative drugs have spasm-reducing effects. These effects are not additive with those of muscle relaxants.

The purpose of sedation

In the context of this book, the purpose of sedation is to allow a procedure, treatment or investigation to be performed. Sedation is therefore not an end in itself, but a process which facilitates another outcome. It is likely that there may be an increased focus on the use of sedation for minor surgical procedures in the UK, as there is an increasing emphasis on the performance of surgery on a day-case basis both in hospitals and in general practitioner surgeries.[6,7]

The duties and competencies of the sedationist will be dealt with in more detail in other chapters. It is vital to remember that the sedationist is present primarily in order to serve the needs of the patient, rather than the requirements of the operator, and the safety of the patient takes priority over the performance of the procedure. Equally, however, there is no point in subjecting the patient to sedation if the desired result (performance of an adequate procedure) is not achievable.

As the first consideration of the sedationist should always be the safety of the patient, the sedationist should ask whether sedation is actually required at all, or whether in fact referral for anaesthesia is the best option. The answer to this question will depend upon multiple factors, including the technicalities of the proposed procedure (e.g. the time taken, the degree of discomfort anticipated, the position the patient may have to adopt, etc.). For example, it has been suggested that although it is more labour and resource intensive, general anaesthesia for MRI scanning in children may result in better-quality images, due to more reliable patient immobility than can be achieved with sedation.[8]

Once the decision has been made to provide sedation, the sedationist must ensure that everything has been done to ensure that the patient is as safe as possible. To achieve this, the sedationist must be certain of what they are aiming to achieve before proceeding. It is suggested that the goals of sedation should always be:

➽ to ensure the patient's safety and welfare
➽ to minimize physical discomfort and pain
➽ to control anxiety, minimise psychological trauma and maximise the potential for amnesia
➽ the control of behaviour and/or movement to allow the safe completion of the procedure
➽ the return of the patient to a state in which safe discharge from medical supervision is possible.

These goals succinctly describe the basis of safe sedation practice.

Alternatives to sedation
Non-pharmacological methods
After consultation with a patient it may be obvious that sedation will not be the best option for their particular case. Other interventions can be considered if the proposed therapeutic intervention is a minor one (e.g. blood sampling, simple tooth extraction, etc.), although anecdotally

techniques such as hypnotism and acupuncture have also been employed for larger surgical procedures.

Increasingly, health practitioners are being informed that patients are 'needle phobic', 'hospital phobic' or 'dental phobic.' This may indicate some real phobia in the medical sense, or some past trauma in relation to medical treatment, or in some cases it may indicate nothing more than a patient preference 'not to have a needle.' It is good practice for the sedationist to see the patient before the procedure, and to develop a professional rapport with them. This will include taking note of any medical history, but also exploring the patient's wishes and beliefs with regard to the treatment they are due to receive. Truly needle- or hospital-phobic patients may not even be able to cross the threshold of the hospital or clinic, and may require a course of therapy before they can even attend for treatment. Alternatively, it may be discovered that a 'phobic' patient has nothing more than a misunderstanding about what is likely to occur. By identifying and addressing such issues, the sedationist may find a way around any fear that the patient has. For example, the author once had to interview a patient who refused cataract surgery under sedation because she believed that her entire eyeball would be removed, polished and then replaced – something she felt that she would never be able to tolerate. When she understood that this was not the case, she happily underwent the procedure using only local anaesthetic.

Behavioural therapy can be particularly important in this context, especially with children. The implementation of so-called 'Saturday Clinics' allows children to attend the ward before they are due to be admitted for elective procedures, familiarises them with the staff and the environment, and gives them an opportunity to ask any questions they wish. Play therapy can assist enormously in reassuring both the child and the parents. During minor procedures such as venepuncture, distraction therapy may avoid the need for sedation altogether.

General anaesthesia

The sedationist should always be aware that general anaesthesia could be the best option for a patient. This may be particularly true when a procedure is likely to be lengthy or require a large degree of immobility, or when it may require a degree of cooperation in an otherwise uncooperative patient (e.g. holding the breath for imaging). Alternatively, if the patient has a serious health problem, or an alarming possible difficulty is discovered at an early stage, the sedationist may recommend that the procedure is performed with an anaesthetist present.

Sedation-related problems

Problems that arise during sedation can be divided into three categories:
- those related to the procedure
- those related to the patient
- those related to the sedation technique used.

Problems related to the procedure include bleeding, pain, the need for immobility, and so on. The effects of these complications can range from a minor inconvenience to the operator, to a major threat to the patient's health (e.g. coronary artery dissection during percutaneous coronary intervention). Problems related to the patient include failure to cooperate, or the exacerbation of an existing medical condition (e.g. angina, asthma). The sedationist must be able to play an active and useful role in stabilising the patient's condition if such difficulties arise.

Problems related to the sedation technique itself fall into three sub-categories. Under-sedation is by far the most common problem. This results in the patient becoming restless or uncooperative because they are not as comfortable as they had been promised they would be. This can result in anxiety, fear and psychological trauma. Under-sedation occurs either because the sedationist has underestimated the amount of drug required to achieve the desired effect, or because the sedationist is afraid of over-sedating the patient.

Over-sedation is much more dangerous to the patient's physical well-being than under-sedation, as it is associated with respiratory depression, airway obstruction, hypoxia, hypercarbia and, in extreme cases, brain damage or death. Over-sedation may not manifest until well into the recovery period, after the treatment has finished. Such severe consequences of over-sedation may be uncommon, but in every series of reported sedation-related deaths, analysis reveals that the great majority of these deaths were preventable. In essence, over-sedation can be a serious hazard, and is often complicated by failure to recognise it and to rescue the patient.

Finally, there may be medication-related problems. These can range from known side-effects of drugs to idiopathic reactions, such as anaphylaxis. There is always a risk that the sedation medications chosen may interact with drugs that the patient is already taking (or with each other, if combinations of sedative drugs are used), producing exaggerated or unanticipated effects. There is also the possibility of drug error, which can result in accidental under-dosage, accidental over-dosage, or the administration of the wrong drug altogether. It is therefore recommended that sedationists should draw up and mix the drugs they are to use themselves, and that every syringe should be properly labelled. The UK has recently adopted a consistent colour-coded system for labelling of anaesthetic drug syringes[9,10] (*see* Table 1.4). If such labels are not available, the sedationist should find another method of ensuring that each drug in each syringe is clearly identifiable.

The clinical example in Box 1.1 illustrates the importance of this last point.

TABLE 1.4 UK standardised pre-printed drug label colours

DRUG TYPE	EXAMPLES	LABEL COLOUR
Anaesthetic induction agents	Propofol	Yellow
	Ketamine	
	Thiopentone	
Opiate analgesics	Morphine	Blue
	Fentanyl	
	Pethidine	
Muscle relaxants	Suxamethonium	Red
	Pancuronium	
	Vecuronium	
	Atracurium	
Hypnotics	Midazolam	Orange
Local anaesthetics	Lignocaine	Grey
	Bupivacaine	

BOX 1.1 The importance of drug labelling

In 2001 an 18-month-old child, J, was admitted to a children's hospital with a heart problem. He was to be taken for a scan, and Nurse A was assigned to escort him. Although she was an experienced children's nurse, Nurse A had no experience of sedation. J was seen by a doctor, and it was decided that sedation would not be necessary. However, ward staff drew up the usual emergency drugs that were taken whenever a child left the ward for a procedure, which included midazolam. Nurse A was told to take these medications with her. None of the syringes were labelled. During the procedure, J became agitated, and Nurse A administered what she believed to be a small dose of midazolam to reduce his anxiety. Unfortunately, what was actually administered was the muscle relaxant vecuronium. Inevitably, J stopped breathing. It was some time before the error became apparent, and by this time J had suffered hypoxic brain damage, from which he died. Nurse A was subsequently found 'not guilty' of manslaughter. She received a caution from the NMC.

Doctor 'at loss' over boy's death; http://news.bbc.co.uk/1/hi/england/merseyside/4333835.stm (accessed 6 July 2007).

www.nmc-uk.org/aDisplayDocument.aspx?DocumentID=2992 (accessed 6 July 2007).

Summary

By properly defining the term 'sedation', we can better understand what can be achieved by the correct utilisation of this technique. It is just as important to understand what cannot be achieved using sedation, as this will help to define a 'scope of practice.' A full understanding of such basic concepts is part of the grounding that every potential sedationist will require in order to develop their competence.

LEARNING POINTS

- Sedation is a technique in which a drug or drugs produce depression of the central nervous system, enabling treatment to be carried out without physical or psychological stress, but during which verbal contact with the patient is maintained.
- Different levels of sedation have been defined, but there are some differences between countries with regard to whether 'deep sedation' is in fact sedation or general anaesthesia.
- It is important that practitioners who are utilising sedation understand the limits of what can be achieved by this technique.
- A sedative drug is likely to have the potential to cause adverse effects on respiratory function.
- The sedationist's first duty is to ensure patient safety.

References

1 American Society of Anesthesiologists. *Continuum of Depth of Sedation. Definition of general anaesthesia and levels of sedation/analgesia* (approved by ASA House of Delegates on 13 October 1999); www.asahg.org/publicationsAndServices/standards/20.htm (accessed 13 April 2007).

2 American Society of Anesthesiologists. *Continuum of Depth of Sedation. Definition of general anaesthesia and levels of sedation/analgesia* (approved by ASA House of Delegates on 13 October 1999, and amended on 27 October 2004); www.asahg.org/publicationsAndServices/standards/20.htm (accessed 13 April 2007).

3 American Society of Anesthesiologists Task Force on Sedation and Analgesia by Non-Anesthesiologists. Practice guidelines for sedation and analgesia by non-anesthesiologists. *Anesthesiology.* 2002; **96:** 1004–17.

4 UK Academy of Medical Royal Colleges and their Faculties. *Implementing and Ensuring Safe Sedation Practice for Healthcare Procedures in Adults;* www.rcoa.ac.uk/docs/safesedationpractice.pdf (accessed 5 July 2007).

5 Runciman WB. Report from the Australian Patient Safety Foundation: Australasian incident monitoring study. *Anaesth Intensive Care.* 1989; **17:** 107–8.

6 NHS Modernisation Agency. *10 High Impact Changes for Service Improvement and Delivery. A guide for NHS leaders.* London: Department of Health; 2004.

7 Department of Health. *Our Health, Our Care, Our Say: making it happen;* www.dh.gov.uk/en/Publicationsandstatistics/Publications/PublicationsPolicyAndGuidance/DH_4139925 (accessed 1 August 2007).

8 Davis C, Razavi R, Baker EJ. Sedation versus general anaesthesia for MRI scanning in children. *Arch Dis Child.* 2000; **83:** 276–9.

9 Association of Anaesthetists Safety Committee. *Syringe Labelling in Critical Care Areas. June 2004 update;* www.rcoa.ac.uk/docs/syringelabels(june).pdf (accessed 1 April 2007).

10 Royal College of Anaesthetists. Syringe labelling in critical care areas. *R Coll Anaesth Bull.* 2003; **19:** 953.

CHAPTER 2

Training in sedation

By defining the skills that a competent sedationist should possess, we can create an outline of an educational and training syllabus through which these abilities can be acquired, maintained and developed. The standards for training suggested in this chapter are derived from several key documents.[1-8] The assumption has been made that the core competencies required for a sedationist of whatever clinical background, in whatever clinical specialty, will be the same. It should be noted that it is UK practice that is referred to, in which deep sedation is regarded as a level of anaesthesia.

Competency in sedation

Competencies for anaesthetists have been well established by professional bodies such as the Royal College of Anaesthetists.[9-12] However, although some formal qualifications and training in sedation are available from some sources (e.g. the Certificate of Dental Sedation Nursing), traditional training for dentists and doctors in this field has been unstructured and haphazard. This is because sedation has been seen as an 'add-on' generalist skill that could best be acquired by experience, rather than by specific training as is the case with anaesthesia. As we have seen from Chapter 1, the states of sedation and anaesthesia are part of a continuum, and it is easy to cross over from one to the other. Therefore there is some requirement for sedationists to share some competencies with anaesthetists. However, although anaesthetic standards and training can guide the skills acquisition of sedationists, the training is not directly transferable. For example, the anaesthetic authorities do not support the concept of *operator-anaesthetist* (i.e. the same practitioner giving the anaesthetic and performing the procedure), whereas the role of *operator-sedationist* has been well established in many other areas of practice, particularly dentistry.

Various attempts have been made to define which particular skills are required to ensure that the sedationist is competent, but such recommendations have essentially remained specialty based, without formal monitored training. As a result, the clinical specialties that have led the way in attempting to create a list of general competencies that should be common to all sedationists, irrespective of background, are anaesthesia and dentistry. Organisations such as the Dental Sedation Teaching Group (www.dstg. co.uk) and the Society for the Advancement of Anaesthesia in Dentistry (www.saaduk.org) have been particularly active in this area.[13]

Core sedationist skills

In order to define a training regime, it is necessary to identify a list of core competencies that need to be addressed. A suggested set of competencies is shown in Table 2.1.

TABLE 2.1 Suggested core competencies for sedationists

GENERAL SKILLS
Communicate effectively with anxious patients.
Obtain an appropriate medical/surgical/anaesthetic/social history, including physical evaluation.
Assess the need for sedation/behavioural management.
Formulate an appropriate treatment plan.
Obtain valid consent.
Give appropriate pre-operative instructions.
Record accurate, concise, clear notes.
Ensure that the environment is safe.
Select and check the appropriate equipment.
Administer supplemental oxygen.
Apply appropriate emergency skills.
Use appropriate airway equipment and support the airway if necessary.
Assess fitness for discharge and provide appropriate post-operative instructions.
Keep a log book, reflect upon practice and identify training needs.
Maintain a caring and professional attitude at all times, including recognition of when assistance is required.

IV SEDATION

Select and prepare all drugs and equipment.

Assess the suitability of veins and perform IV cannulation.

Recognise extravascular injection.

Titrate the drug to the required level of sedation.

INHALATIONAL SEDATION

Check machine and scavenging.

Connect the breathing system and check the mask.

Titrate sedation as necessary.

MONITORING

Select and use appropriate monitoring, and make decisions and treat the patient on the basis of derived data.

SEDATION-RELATED COMPLICATIONS

Recognise and respond to sedation-related complications (e.g. over- or under-sedation, respiratory depression, airway obstruction, etc.) appropriately.

Remain calm, decisive and purposeful during emergencies.

Recognise and participate in the treatment of procedure-related complications (e.g. bleeding).

Recognise and participate in the treatment of any other possible emergency (e.g. anaphylaxis, cardiac arrest, local anaesthetic toxicity).

Categorisation of skills

Having successfully defined a set of sedationist skills, it is then possible to delineate how they should be obtained, and to what standard.

These skills can be classified into the following categories:

➼ the ability to appropriately assess and select patients

➼ the ability to formulate and implement an appropriate treatment plan

➼ the ability to recognise and deal with emergency situations.

The ability to appropriately assess and select patients

The sedationist is accountable for their own actions, and so as an independent practitioner they must take ownership of their own practice. This means that it is their own responsibility to acquire the knowledge that will allow them to practise their craft safely. Sedationists must therefore possess the ability to ensure that the patient has been appropriately selected to undergo sedation. In many departments where sedation is commonly used, the patient may have passed through a thorough pre-operative selection process, including a history, examination and series of appropriate investigations. However, the sedationist must be sure in their own mind that sedation is an appropriate technique for this particular patient, and should not embark upon a procedure unless they are totally satisfied that this is the case. The sedationist must therefore be able to perform their own assessment.

Whether a patient is suitable for sedation will depend upon many factors, including the type of procedure to be performed, the patient's state of health, the facilities available, and so on. As basic as it seems, the patient must understand what is meant by sedation, and must be willing to cooperate with the procedure. For example, a planned inhalational technique may induce panic in a claustrophobic patient when a face mask is applied.

The sedationist should ensure that he or she is familiar with the patient's history from the notes, and then briefly check that no different or new symptoms have occurred since the previous assessment. Cardiac and respiratory symptoms are particularly relevant, but other health problems can also be important. A reasonable history will include questions about the patient's allergies, medications and last meal. The latter is particularly controversial as, in contrast to the situation with anaesthesia, some authorities would allow patients to eat or drink before sedation is given electively, possibly increasing the risk of aspiration. Previous operations may also be of relevance. For example, it is not usual to place a drip in the arm of a patient on the same side as a previous axillary lymph node clearance for breast cancer, in case tissue oedema occurs. A brief history relating to previous anaesthetics or sedatives should also be obtained (*see* Box 2.1).

BOX 2.1 The importance of a family history

A young girl, X, presented for a minor surgical procedure. When she was seen by the anaesthetist, a large number of relatives were present. On questioning about previous anaesthetics, it became clear that a first-degree relative had been admitted to Intensive Care some years previously following an 'allergy to anaesthesia.' The details were vague, but the anaesthetist managed to discuss this with X's grandmother, who stated that the events had occurred over 20 years ago, and that the relative in question had taken 'a long time to breathe.' The anaesthetist provisionally diagnosed scoline apnoea, and adjusted the anaesthetic technique accordingly. The diagnosis was later confirmed, and the rest of the family were subsequently tested for the condition.

Some of the issues relevant to the history of previous anaesthetics or sedatives are listed in Table 2.2.

TABLE 2.2 Issues relevant to the history of previous anaesthetics or sedatives

QUESTIONS RELEVANT TO THE HISTORY OF PREVIOUS ANAESTHETICS OR SEDATIVES	RELEVANCE
Has the patient had previous sedation or anaesthesia? When did these other procedures occur? At what facility did they occur?	If the notes of these procedures are available, they will answer many questions with regard to previous episodes, including what drugs were administered, and any difficulties that arose. It may be possible to acquire this information directly from the patient's general practitioner, or the other facility.
Were there any difficulties or complications related to the anaesthetics?	Adverse reactions to anaesthetics, airway difficulties, difficulties in venous access, etc.
Were there any other adverse events in relation to these episodes?	Cardiovascular events, respiratory events, allergies, exacerbations of underlying illnesses, etc.
Does the patient have any allergies?	Drugs which may be given to which the patient is allergic (e.g. antibiotics) should be identified, as should the nature of the resultant 'allergy.'
Have any relatives had an adverse reaction to an anaesthetic?	Some anaesthetic reactions run in families (e.g. malignant hyperpyrexia, scoline apnoea). Barbiturates and some local anaesthetics are contraindicated in patients with porphyria.

After taking a brief history, a relevant physical examination should be performed. Normally, little more than examination of the cardiovascular and respiratory system is necessary. However, other physiological systems may require examination if the history suggests that there may be a problem. The oral cavity and airway may be particularly relevant in this regard. The sedationist should ensure that all relevant tests have been performed, and that they have been appropriately interpreted.

The tests that should be performed prior to undergoing anaesthesia, surgery or sedation will vary from patient to patient depending upon their ASA (American Society of Anesthesiologists) status (*see* page 27), the proposed procedure, and the occurrence of any intermittent illnesses. These have been summarised by the National Institute for Health and Clinical Excellence (NICE)[14] in the UK. Although this guidance is aimed at patients undergoing anaesthesia for surgical procedures, there is no evidence to suggest that patients undergoing procedures under sedation need to be investigated any less thoroughly.

It is also important to ensure that the environment is an appropriate one for performing the procedure. There may be a variety of reasons why the patient can undergo sedation for the procedure safely, but not in the available facility, in which case other arrangements should be made.[15,16]

Social factors are also an important issue for consideration. Patients undergoing procedures under sedation in hospital may be doing so on an outpatient or day-case basis, being discharged home later. Staff, including the sedationist, should ensure that the social circumstances at home will allow the safe discharge of the patient.

Once the sedationist has considered all of these factors, they can make an informed decision as to whether it is appropriate to proceed with sedation. If there is any doubt as to the suitability of the patient, the sedationist is responsible for taking action, which may include deferring the patient's treatment.

The ability to formulate and implement an appropriate treatment plan

Based upon their knowledge of the patient's health and history, the facilities available, and the procedure to be performed, the sedationist can decide upon an appropriate treatment plan. This plan will include not only which sedative agent will be given, but how the patient will be monitored, and the 'back-up' plan should the sedation not achieve the desired effect. In addition, it should include the actions that will be taken if an emergency arises.

There are broadly three types of sedation technique, namely *inhalational*, *gastrointestinal/mucosal* and *intravenous* sedation. Gastrointestinal/mucosal techniques usually involve the administration of a drug orally, although other routes have also been used. The inhalational and intravenous routes allow the drug dose to be titrated against the response of the patient, so are more predictable and manageable. These techniques are discussed in more detail in Chapters 5, 6, 8 and 9.

The level of sedation required will depend upon the surgical procedure or investigation proposed. Dental extractions and MRI scanning may require only anxiolysis in most adult patients, but conscious sedation may be required in particularly nervous individuals. Other factors may also determine whether sedation is required. For example, conscious sedation is generally required for endoscopic sigmoidoscopies, not only to reduce anxiety, but also to impair the patient's recollection of what is a rather undignified procedure.

The sedationist must also be able to plan which type of monitoring is required, and be able to record the progress of the sedation properly. In addition, there is a responsibility to ensure that the treatment is recorded correctly in the patient records. These duties are discussed further in Chapters 4 and 6.

The sedationist has a duty to ensure that the environment in which the procedure is to occur is appropriate. The facilities available will vary in different environments, and the sedationist must be satisfied that they achieve nationally and locally defined standards. The sedationist has shared responsibility with the organisation and the other members of the team caring for the patient in this regard, but has personal responsibility for the drugs and equipment that are being utilised. In addition, it is important to ensure that the available staff have the appropriate skills. These responsibilities are defined in Chapters 4, 5 and 6.

The ability to recognise and deal with emergency situations

The sedationist is responsible for the safety of the patient, and must therefore be able to recognise when a problem has arisen, and to take appropriate action to alleviate the emergency until help arrives. Emergencies which can affect the safety of the patient can be classified as arising from three main sources.

Complications arising from the procedure that is being performed

Every therapeutic or investigative procedure carries a risk of complications, many of which will be of minor significance. However, some problems will have major implications with regard to either the ability to perform the procedure, or the safety of the patient. For example, if a claustrophobic patient has a panic attack while undergoing MRI scanning, this will prevent the scan being performed, and may have psychological sequelae, but may not cause the patient physical harm. However, a pneumothorax created during the insertion of a central line may require emergency treatment. The common complications of surgical procedures that can arise during the act of sedation include bleeding, pain, technical difficulty and damage to surrounding tissues. The operator will be responsible for dealing with these issues, but the sedationist must be able to assist in their resolution and management (e.g. by ensuring that assistance is summoned, reassuring the patient, administering analgesia, etc.).

If diathermy is being used during the procedure, all staff should be aware of the possible fire risk, particularly if alcohol-based skin cleansers are used. Equally, staff should know what action to take in the unlikely event of electrocution occurring.

Complications arising from the sedation or analgesia

Complications arising from drug treatment can include known side-effects, or reactions that are personal to a particular patient (e.g. allergy). The commonest hazardous side-effect of the administration of sedative drugs and analgesics is over-sedation, with consequent risk to the airway, and resultant hypoxia. The sedationist must be able to monitor the patient appropriately, and act in a timely manner if airway compromise is suspected. This may include calling for assistance, administering more oxygen, supporting the airway, or even ventilating the patient using airway adjuncts. The sedationist should also be able to detect and handle the complications related to drugs that are administered by the operator, such as local anaesthetic agents.

Patient-related complications

These include complications arising from any illnesses of the patient. For example, diabetic patients may become hypo- or hyperglycaemic, patients with epilepsy could have a seizure, and patients with ischaemic heart disease could have an angina attack or a myocardial infarction. The sedationist should be aware of these potential hazards and should be able to commence supportive treatment as necessary. It is recommended that staff are appropriately trained in cardiopulmonary resuscitation (CPR).

Formal training

Although it is always possible to acquire knowledge and skills by attending dedicated courses in a given subject, sedation is a practical subject that is best learned by 'doing.' Practical training in sedation should occur in a controlled and supervised manner as part of a well-defined curriculum. Unfortunately, many medical training schemes do not have any provision for formal training in practical sedation. However, some work on how these essential skills should be acquired has been done in other areas. It is assumed that the trainee sedationist will be undergoing formal supervision, and will be subject to assessment both by logbook and by formal structured observation. Table 2.3 summarises the main recommendations made by the Dental Sedation Teachers Group (DSTG).

TABLE 2.3 DSTG training recommendations for sedation in dentistry

Patient assessment: the trainee should be supervised and noted as competent in 5 cases.

Assessment includes history taking, examination skills, ordering and interpretation of tests, understanding of common illnesses and effects of sedation in relation to these, and assessment of potential hazards such as allergies, medications, substance abuse and oral history of tobacco substance abuse. It also includes physical examination, ordering appropriate laboratory tests, obtaining consent and discussion of risks.

Inhalational sedation: supervised and assessed in 10 cases.

Includes airway assessment, use of pulse oximeter, ability to support airway and use bag and mask, etc., recording of appropriate observations, and use of appropriate monitoring.

Intravenous sedation: supervised and assessed in a further 20 cases.

Includes intravenous line insertion, and choice and use of drugs.

Clinical governance

A key element of safe practice is ensuring that the system within which one is working is constantly developing and improving. This concept can be defined by the term 'clinical governance', which was introduced into UK medical terminology in the late 1990s. It is defined as 'a framework through which healthcare organisations are accountable for continuously improving the quality of their services and safeguarding high standards of care by creating an environment in which excellence in clinical care will flourish.'[17–19]

The philosophy of clinical governance suggests that it is the responsibility of all staff to ensure that errors and faults are reported and corrected, and a further responsibility is to ensure that good practices are identified and built upon. The aim is to ensure that the healthcare organisation has a memory for good practice, and avoids repeating past mistakes.[20] Clinical audit is a key part of this process. Audit can be defined as 'a quality improvement process that seeks to improve patient care and outcomes through systematic review of care against explicit criteria and the implementation of change.'[21] In simple terms, an individual or organisation can define a quality standard to which to work, and can then examine the results to see whether this is being achieved. If it is not, the system is changed and the audit is then re-performed to see whether improvement has resulted. This process of 'closing the audit loop', whereby audit becomes a continuous cycle of examination and improvement, can apply to personal as well as organisational development.

Audit of personal development has two aspects. The first is an audit of personal clinical practice. At its simplest, this will be a mere record of clinical cases performed. However, there is more to personal audit than recording a volume of cases completed. It is far more meaningful for the purposes of training to also record details of difficult or unusual cases which, when reflected upon, may lead to changes in the approach to similar issues in future. The Dental Sedation Teachers Group has published a useful example of such a logbook on its website.[22]

It is also important for individuals to record academic activity which relates to their everyday practice. It is generally accepted that the educational courses that one attends should for the most part reflect one's clinical work. For example, an individual working mainly with children should ensure that they participate in activities that will support their knowledge and work in this field.

Practitioners should ensure that the systems within which they work are also subjected to regular scrutiny. Although the healthcare organisation has responsibility for confirming the overall standards of the equipment, environment and personnel available, the individuals concerned have a duty to ensure that the systems within which they are working function appropriately at all times. This includes ensuring that problems are promptly reported to a higher authority through the appropriate mechanism. It is also important that the global function of a department is monitored. This will include analysing not only the practice of individuals providing a particular service, but also the activities of the service as a whole. Such activity can be beneficial to the organisation, to the individual practitioner and to patients. Various professional bodies can provide information about the efficiency of services. The Royal College of Anaesthetists publishes a regularly updated compendium of 'audit recipes' which can be very useful in this context.[23]

Summary

Although sedation is a practical subject, training should only take place in a controlled, supervised environment as part of a formal training scheme. All procedures should be carried out under the direct supervision of a suitably trained sedationist. It is recommended that the sedationist possesses the appropriate skills to allow them to practise in the interests of the patient independently, without instruction from or direct supervision by the operator/surgeon. If the sedationist is participating in the performance of the procedure or investigation, the monitoring of the patient must be delegated to an appropriately trained individual, although the operator-sedationist is ultimately responsible for the safety of both the sedation techniques and the procedure itself. Sedationists will have some skills in common with anaesthetists. The syllabus outlined above and examined in detail in the rest of this book has been derived from a large number of sources. Although practices may differ between specialties, the common theme of all the reports and papers is that sedation is not a pastime for the occasional practitioner. Both training and practice will need to be subjected to regular audit in order to ensure that standards are maintained.

LEARNING POINTS

- Sedation is used in many clinical scenarios.
- The core competencies for sedationists should be common to all practitioners, irrespective of background.
- Training in sedation will have features in common with anaesthetic training, but sedationists do not need to have undergone full anaesthetic training.

References

1 Dental Sedation Teachers Group. *Sedation in Dentistry: undergraduate training guidelines for teachers;* www.dstg.co.uk/teaching (accessed 1 July 2007).

2 Dental Sedation Teachers Group. *Sedation in Dentistry: the competent graduate;* www.dstg.co.uk/teaching/competent-graduate/ (accessed 1 July 2007).

3 Dental Sedation Teachers Group. *Training for Safe Practice in Advanced Sedation Techniques for Adult Patients;* www.dstg.co.uk/teaching/advanced-sedation (accessed 25 June 2007).

4 Dental Sedation Teachers Group. *Training in Conscious Sedation for Dentistry;* www.dstg.co.uk/teaching (accessed 24 May 2007).

5 European Academy of Paediatric Dentistry. Curriculum guidelines for education and training in paediatric dentistry. *Int J Paediatr Dent.* 1997; **7**: 273–81.

6 Royal College of Surgeons of England. *Report of the Working Party on Guidelines for Sedation by Non-Anaesthetists;* www.rcseng.ac.uk/rcseng/content/publications/docs/publication.2005-09-01.1561369700 (accessed 23 February 2007).

7 Royal College of Nursing. *Day Surgery Information. Managing patients undergoing sedation;* www.rcn.org.uk/publications/pdf/daysurgery_sedation.pdf (accessed 21 July 2007).

8 Scottish Dental Clinical Effectiveness Programme. *Conscious Sedation in Dentistry. Dental clinical guidance;* www.scottishdental.org/cep/docs/Concious_Sedation_in_Dentistry.pdf (accessed 12 June 2007).

9 Royal College of Anaesthetists. *CCT in Anaesthesia. I. General principles. A manual for trainees and trainers;* www.rcoa.ac.uk/docs/CCTpti.pdf (accessed 30 July 2007).

10 Royal College of Anaesthetists. *CCT in Anaesthesia. II. Competency-based basic level*

(ST Years 1 and 2) training and assessment. A manual for trainees and trainers; www.rcoa.ac.uk/docs/CCTptii.pdf (accessed 29 July 2007).

11 Royal College of Anaesthetists. *CCT in Anaesthesia. III. Competency-based intermediate level (Years 3 and 4) training and assessment. A manual for trainees and trainers;* www.rcoa.ac.uk/docs/CCTptiii.pdf (accessed 28 July 2007).

12 Royal College of Anaesthetists. *CCT in Anaesthesia. IV. Competency-based higher and advanced level (Years 5, 6 and 7) training and assessment. A manual for trainees and trainers;* www.rcoa.ac.uk/docs/CCTptiv.pdf (accessed 29 July 2007).

13 Debuse D. Society for the Advancement of Anaesthesia in Dentistry (SAAD). *Anaesthesia News.* 2007; **241:** 32–3.

14 National Institute for Health and Clinical Excellence. *The Use of Routine Preoperative Tests for Elective Surgery;* http://guidance.nice.org.uk/CG3/?c=296725 (accessed 22 February 2007).

15 Ni KM, Watts JC. Day-case surgery in an isolated unit may require more stringent selection of cases. *Anaesthesia.* 2001; **56:** 485–6.

16 Watts J, Ni K. Obesity and day-case surgery in an isolated unit. *Anaesthesia.* 2002; **57:** 290–91.

17 Scally G, Donaldson LJ. Clinical governance and the drive for quality improvement in the new NHS in England. *BMJ.* 1998; **317:** 61–5; www.bmj.com/cgi/content/full/317/7150/61 (accessed 16 August 2007).

18 Department of Health. *The New NHS: modern, dependable;* www.archive.official-documents.co.uk/document/doh/newnhs/contents.htm (accessed 16 August 2007).

19 Department of Health. *A First Class Service: quality in the new NHS;* www.dh.gov.uk/en/Publicationsandstatistics/Publications/PublicationsPolicyAndGuidance/DH_4006902 (accessed 16 August 2007).

20 Department of Health. *Building a Safer NHS for Patients: implementing an organisation with a memory;* www.dh.gov.uk/en/Publicationsandstatistics/Publications/PublicationsPolicyAndGuidance/DH_4006525 (accessed 16 August 2007).

21 National Institute for Clinical Excellence. *Principles for Best Practice in Clinical Audit;* www.nice.org.uk/page.aspx?o=29058 (accessed 16 August 2007).

22 Dental Sedation Teachers Group. *Logbook of Clinical Experience in Conscious Sedation;* www.dstg.co.uk/teaching/logbook/sedationlogbook.doc (accessed 16 August 2007).

23 Colvin JR, editor. *Raising the Standard. A compendium of audit recipes for continuous quality improvement in anaesthesia.* 2nd ed; www.rcoa.ac.uk/index.asp?PageID=125 (accessed 17 September 2007).

CHAPTER 3

Patient assessment and selection

Any medical, nursing or surgical intervention must be performed in the best interests of the patient. This means that the healthcare professional must use their judgement to decide whether the procedure is more likely to benefit than harm the patient. Key information that the healthcare professional needs to acquire before they can make this assessment includes the patient's state of health, and how this may affect or be affected by the proposed treatment. Therefore a central skill for the sedationist is the ability to assess the patient's suitability for undergoing the proposed treatment. It is in no one's interest for a patient to undergo a successful procedure from which they have no chance of surviving to get benefit.

The concept of risk

No one can reduce the risk arising from medical treatment to 'zero', because medical treatment of any kind is not a neutral, risk-free act. The most that can be hoped for is that the level of risk is reduced as much as possible by controlling the factors that can safely be limited in the time available. A good risk analogy would be crossing a road. Crossing a road is a dangerous activity, but the risk related to the act will depend upon many factors, such as the dimensions of the road itself, the speed of movement of the pedestrian, and the density and velocity of traffic. However, there may also be unpredictable hazards that are not so obvious, but which will also need to be navigated (e.g. loose manhole covers, potholes, etc.). It can be seen from this analogy that the sedationist has a key role in getting the patient 'across the road', and therefore needs to be able to identify and minimise preventable risks.

Risks related to medical procedures

The risks to a patient with regard to a procedure or treatment are twofold:

➡ the risks related to the procedure itself:
  — general risks related to any procedure (e.g. bleeding, infection, side-effects)
  — specific risks related to a particular procedure (e.g. bowel perforation, pneumothorax, etc.)
  — risks related to the sedation or anaesthesia necessary to allow the procedure to take place

➡ the risks related to the patient's underlying health.

The sedationist needs to take into consideration all of these factors before embarking on their treatment of the patient. After a proper assessment, which will involve a full history, a relevant examination and appropriate investigations, the sedationist must formulate a treatment plan that is safe, but which accommodates the wishes of the patient (where possible) as well as the needs of the operator. The sedationist must bear in mind that they have a duty to be the patient's advocate, and that they must advise the patient appropriately at all times. For example, not all patients will be suitable for the proposed treatment, and not all patients will be suitable for the proposed sedation.

The correct treatment plan may well be to decide that the patient will not benefit from the proposed procedure, and to arrange alternative treatment.

Patient-related factors

Assessment of a patient's suitability for sedation will include an estimate of their current health status, based upon information gleaned from the history, examination and available investigation results.

For many years, anaesthetists have been classifying patients according to their ASA (American Society of Anesthesiologists) grade (*see* Table 3.1). The ASA system is a ubiquitous way of classifying the patient crudely in terms of their risk, based upon the perceived debility resulting from any illness from which they may be suffering. The higher the ASA grade, the more unwell the patient is, and so the higher the risk.[1,2] For example, a patient may be described by anaesthetists as 'ASA 1' or 'ASA 4.' In addition, the suffix 'E' is added if the patient is an emergency case (e.g. 'ASA 3 E').

The system is not perfect. It is supposed to classify the patient according to their ASA grade when they are 'well', which may bear no relation to their grade when they are ill. In addition, there are several categories of illness which do not fit easily into the grading provided. For example, patients with psychiatric illness may be physically well, but are often subjected to poly-pharmacy, utilising drugs with a broad range of side-effects; and pregnant women are at substantially greater risk of morbidity due to physiological changes than their non-pregnant counterparts. Furthermore, the effects of ageing on ASA grading have not been clearly elucidated. This inevitably leads to some inter-observer variability in scoring.

TABLE 3.1 The ASA Grading System

GRADE	DEFINITION	DESCRIPTION	ESTIMATED ASSOCIATED MORTALITY
1	A fit and well patient with no illnesses	Normal healthy adult	0–0.3%
2	A patient with an illness that is well controlled, and does not interfere with their normal activities	Mild asthma, well controlled diabetes, occasional angina, etc.	0.3–1.4%
3	A patient with an illness that is not well controlled, or who has more than one illness, which does affect their normal activities	Moderate asthma, poorly controlled diabetes, controlled heart failure	1.8–5.4%
4	A patient who has an illness, or more than one illness, which is a constant threat to their life	Severe heart failure, severe ischaemic heart disease, etc.	7.8–25.9%
5	A moribund patient who may not survive without intervention	Trauma victim, major haemorrhage, etc.	9.4–57.8%

The scheme does therefore have its limitations and its critics. However, it has the advantage of being a system that is easily understood and applied. As such it is often used to filter patients out from undergoing certain procedures in certain environments. For example, a local guideline might suggest that an isolated endoscopy unit should only be used for patients who are undergoing elective procedures and are ASA grade 2 or lower, whereas if the unit was part of a main hospital with full support facilities it might be decided that the suite was suitable for the use of patients who are ASA grade 3 and are undergoing emergency procedures. It must be remembered that anaesthetists tend to use this system as a general risk assessment tool, whereas it was originally designed only for use with surgical patients.

Patient assessment

The sedationist must have the time and facilities available to see and assess the patients themselves before the operation or procedure takes place. This not only allows an appropriate rapport to be established with the patient, but it also enables the sedationist to perform an appropriate risk assessment.

Most modern health facilities will have established 'pre-operative assessment' procedures for patients who are listed for surgical treatment. Often, in the case of surgical patients, this will be run from a specific clinic. Whatever system is adopted locally, this should mean that by the time the sedationist sees the patient, all of the relevant information which is necessary for them to make a decision is available. This will include details of the proposed procedure, a 'first sieve' of any relevant medical history, and the results of appropriate investigations. However, the sedationist must base their decisions and actions upon their own assessment of the patient, taking into account – but not solely relying upon – information provided by others. For example, it is possible that between the visit to the pre-operative assessment clinic and the sedationist's assessment, the patient may have developed new symptoms (e.g. more frequent angina, new shortness of breath, etc.).

The sedationist should therefore be able to take an appropriate history (including any allergies, medications, time of last meal, and relevant medical symptoms), perform an appropriate examination (e.g. airway assessment, cardiovascular system, etc.), and request and interpret appropriate tests (e.g. blood results, X-rays, echocardiograms, etc.). They must then be able to correlate this information and draw a conclusion about the suitability of the patient. The essential question that the sedationist must be able to answer is whether the patient's physiological condition is the best that can reasonably be achieved and, if so, whether they are suitable for the proposed procedure (*see* Box 3.1).

> **BOX 3.1 The importance of a good pre-operative assessment**
>
> A patient, Z, presented for a major surgical procedure, having undergone several minor operations in the recent past. His blood clotting time had been tested at the pre-operative assessment clinic the day before, and was found to be abnormal. The anaesthetist discussed this with the patient, but no history of unusual bleeding was elicited. The test was repeated, and again the clotting time was confirmed to be prolonged. The operation was postponed while further information was sought. Z's parents attended

the next consultation with the anaesthetist, and were questioned about any bleeding tendency in the family. It was discovered that Z's siblings and distant relatives displayed characteristics of an undiagnosed bleeding disorder.

A diagnosis of von Willebrand's disease was later confirmed, and surgery took place under the cover of appropriately administered clotting factors.

The answer will depend upon many factors, including the urgency of the need for the procedure. However, if there is any doubt, serious thought must be given to the possibility of postponing the treatment. This is not always possible, particularly in the case of an evolving time-dependent pathology that requires urgent treatment, such as percutaneous coronary intervention (PCI) angiography, or colonoscopy to investigate a possible cancer.

The patient's medical condition

It is beyond the scope of this book to discuss every possible medical problem at length. However, common conditions and issues are described below in relation to the clinical systems affected.

Age

Age is an independent risk factor for any medical intervention, and so it is to be expected that the elderly will be more vulnerable to complications (*see* Chapter 8). The changes of ageing mean that the elderly patient has reduced 'physiological reserve' if problems arise. They are also more sensitive to the effects of drugs, and doses may need to be adjusted appropriately. Paediatric patients also present additional challenges to the sedationist (*see* Chapter 7).

Respiratory problems
Airway assessment
The sedationist must bear in mind that there is only a fine line between levels of conscious sedation and general anaesthesia, and that there is always a possibility that they may have to intervene if the patient's airway becomes compromised. It is therefore essential that they have a clear understanding of proper airway assessment. 'Airway assessment' means that the sedationist has considered carefully whether there will be any difficulties in supporting the patient's ventilation (up to and including intubation of the trachea) if a problem arises. At its very simplest, this will include an assessment of mouth opening, jaw movement, neck mobility and dentition. Anaesthetists use

the Mallampati grading system to assess the view seen at mouth opening. The sedationist sits opposite the patient and assesses what structures can be seen when the patient has their mouth fully open. A good view of all pharyngeal structures is Mallampati grade 1, whereas a grade 4 view is one in which only the palate can be seen. Higher grades of view are associated with difficulty in viewing the vocal cords at laryngoscopy, and therefore difficulties in intubation, although it should be borne in mind that in an emergency situation it is not always necessary to intubate the trachea. However, it *is* always necessary to maintain oxygenation, and this may require the use of airway adjuncts, which require oral or nasal insertion. If a patient can open their mouth to three fingers' width, it should be easy to insert an oral airway if required. Dentition should be examined for any loose or crumbly teeth which could be displaced and become a potential hazard. A full range of neck movements means that the head can be easily manipulated into optimum airway position. On the other hand, a thin wasted face, a chubby face or a beard may mean that there could be difficulty in holding a face mask in place. A deviated nasal septum can make nasopharyngeal airway insertion difficult.

Anticipated airway difficulty may necessitate a formal anaesthetic presence.

Smoking

Smoking is a general risk factor for many cardiovascular and respiratory diseases, as increased mucus production and reduced clearance can lead to areas of atelectasis (lung collapse). Atelectasis may predispose to post-procedure chest problems. In the elderly, atelectasis may occur even in the semi-recumbent position. There is some debate as to how long before surgery an individual must stop smoking for this risk to decrease significantly.

Asthma

Well controlled asthma should not be a problem during the procedure unless the patient comes into contact with a stimulus that could cause bronchospasm. A careful allergy history is necessary. Poorly controlled asthma should be optimised before a procedure takes place. The means for treating an asthma attack must be available.

Respiratory tract infection

Ideally, the patient should be free from any respiratory tract infection. There may be occasions when this is not possible (e.g. investigation of bronchiectasis), but the presence of a respiratory tract infection predisposes the patient to respiratory complications of varying severity, especially if the respiratory tract is to be subject to instrumentation.

Cardiovascular problems

There are very few justifications for proceeding with sedation and intervention if the patient is suffering from unstable or uncontrolled ischaemic heart disease, unless the purpose of these interventions is to alleviate or treat the underlying cardiac disorder.

The presence of severe heart disease is a major risk factor for predicting death after non-coronary surgery. The Goldman score (*see* Table 3.2) is a commonly used risk assessment system.

TABLE 3.2 The Goldman cardiac risk index

RISK FACTOR	CRITERIA	POINTS
History	Age > 70 years	5
	Heart attack less than 6 months previously	10
Examination	Signs of heart failure (gallop rhythm, raised jugular venous pressure)	11
	Important stenotic valve disease	3
ECG	Any rhythm other than sinus or premature atrial complexes	7
	More than 5 premature ventricular complexes/ minute at any time prior to procedure	7
Status	Blood gases: low oxygen, high carbon dioxide	3
	Low potassium, low bicarbonate	
	Signs of renal impairment	
	Signs of chronic liver disease	
	Patient bedridden due to non-cardiac causes	
Operation	Intra-abdominal, intra-thoracic, aortic	3
	Emergency	4
Maximum possible score		53

SCORE	RISK OF LIFE-THREATENING COMPLICATIONS (%)	RISK OF DEATH (%)
0–5	0.7	0.2
6–12	5	1.5
13–25	11	2.3
26–53	22	56

For example, a 75-year-old man who was undergoing an endoscopy to investigate mild anaemia and heartburn, and who had atrial fibrillation, would have a score of 12, indicating that he was at fairly low risk. However, if he was in heart failure from the associated anaemia, he would score up to 23, and his risk of death from the procedure would therefore be nearly doubled. Other more refined or further adapted tests also exist, not all of which agree with each other in every detail. Such assessment scales are merely tools, and clinical staff must use their skill and judgement in interpreting them and how they apply to their patient. Unstable ischaemic heart disease, unstable cardiac rhythm and signs of heart failure are associated with a very high risk of peri-procedure cardiac complications.

In addition, one must consider how the presence of cardiac pacing devices may be affected by the surgical procedure, especially if diathermy is used. Pacemakers are designed to maintain the cardiac rhythm, and hence cardiac output, and are inserted for a wide variety of reasons. They should be regularly checked to ensure that they are continuing to function correctly. Patients who have these devices usually carry a card which contains all of the information necessary to make an assessment of their function or, failing that, information that will enable the assessor to access a database about the pacemaker in question. Modern pacemakers are very sophisticated, and one cannot assume that the indiscriminate use of a magnet will switch the pacemaker into a safe mode. In addition, *implantable cardiac defibrillators (ICDs)* may be activated by surgical diathermy, with disastrous consequences. If in doubt, contact the patient's cardiology centre for advice.

TABLE 3.3 Duration of antiplatelet therapy and recommended delays in non-cardiac, non-urgent surgery following cardiac interventions

CARDIAC INTERVENTION	DURATION OF ANTIPLATELET THERAPY	DELAY IN NON-URGENT SURGERY
Coronary artery dilatation	2–4 weeks	Vital surgery only: 2–4 weeks
Percutaneous coronary intervention and bare metal stent	4–6 weeks	Vital surgery: > 6 weeks Elective surgery: > 3 months
Percutaneous coronary intervention and drug-eluting stent	12 months	Elective surgery: > 12 months

Increasing numbers of patients are undergoing coronary artery stenting during angiography in order to treat symptomatic ischaemic heart disease, as an alternative to coronary artery bypass grafting (CABG). The sedationist should be alert to the fact that the presence of these stents can significantly increase the likelihood of a serious cardiac event occurring during a non-cardiac treatment or investigation. For this reason it is recommended that any non-urgent surgery is delayed after stent placement (*see* Table 3.3). In addition, patients will remain on antiplatelet medication for some time after a stent has been placed, in order to reduce the possibility of a secondary coronary thrombosis. However, this medication may significantly increase the likelihood of bleeding occurring during treatment. The sedationist should refer to local guidelines when faced with such a patient.[3]

Central nervous system problems

Epilepsy is a common neurological disorder, but it should be appreciated that every patient's symptoms will be unique. The pattern of the patient's seizures, including any heralding aura, must be elicited.[4] The stress of undergoing a medical procedure may be enough to trigger a seizure. If a fit is triggered, this could have an adverse effect on the patient's activities, such as their legal ability to drive, which in turn could have consequences for their employment. Drugs which may lower the seizure threshold, thereby possibly precipitating a fit, should be avoided. Drug doses may need to be modified, as anti-epileptic medication may increase liver metabolism. Sedationists will need to understand how to detect and treat epileptic symptoms.

Movement disorders such as parkinsonism may not be modified by sedation. The presence of a tremor, or rigidity, may seriously impair the ability to perform the planned procedure. If a completely motionless patient is required, general anaesthesia may be the better option.

If the patient is confused or suffering from dementia, a general anaesthetic may be necessary. An uncooperative patient is an indication to abandon the procedure. Paradoxical stimulation may occur following the administration of sedatives, and this again may mean that cancellation and future general anaesthesia is the best option. It is not permissible to forcibly restrain a patient in order to perform a procedure, as this may lead to physical harm (of the staff as well as the patient), and could be regarded as a battery under the law.

A past history of stroke means that the patient is at increased risk of a further cerebrovascular accident in the future. However, it is difficult to clarify this risk, as it does not seem to vary with time from the initial incident, or with factors such as the severity of the previous episode.

Patients may present for procedures (such as scans) in relation to intracranial pathology. This is a field best left to specialist practitioners. If there is any suggestion of raised intracranial pressure (such as a reduced Glasgow Coma Scale score), sedation is contraindicated.

Gastrointestinal problems

The presence of significant heartburn can indicate an increased risk of aspiration during a procedure, with consequent respiratory problems. Symptoms such as recurrent reflux on bending, or while lying in bed at night, or a chronic nocturnal cough, or the presence of a hiatus hernia may indicate the presence of an incompetent lower oesophageal sphincter. This may require the administration of pre-operative antacid medication.

Diabetes is a common disorder of adults and children. As a general rule, operating-theatre practice is that diabetic patients should be fasted like any other patient, but their diabetic medication should be omitted until they are able to take food and fluids orally again. It is sensible to assume that their treatment should take place at the beginning of the morning, or at the beginning of the afternoon session if possible, so that there is ample opportunity to monitor their blood sugar levels before possible discharge from hospital. Diabetics with poor control, those undergoing lengthy procedures and those undergoing procedures which may require prolonged fasting may need to be placed on an intravenous insulin/dextrose/potassium regime in order to control their blood sugar levels. Every organisation should have a local guideline on the management of diabetic patients.

Gastrointestinal bleeding can be torrential, and patients presenting for emergency endoscopy can be in circulatory shock. There is a large potential for occult bleeding, and the stomach may contain a large volume of blood. Consequently there is an increased risk of aspiration in these patients.

Genitourinary problems

Some medications, including sedatives, analgesics and their adjuncts, may predispose to difficulty in passing water even during a brief hospital stay, especially if the patient has a history of prostatism. This may require catheterisation to resolve the problem in the short term.

Since many drugs are excreted via the kidneys, caution should be exercised in the presence of kidney impairment or renal failure. Venous access in renal patients is likely to be difficult. The insertion of cannulae into arms containing arteriovenous shunts for dialysis should be avoided, as damage to the shunt can result in torrential haemorrhage, or require surgery for the formation of a new shunt. Some authorities have recommended that the arm veins in renal patients should not be used at all, but should be preserved for future arteriovenous shunt formation.

Obesity

Clinically obese patients are more at risk of complications of many types, including bleeding, deep vein thrombosis, and infection. Obtaining venous access can be problematic, and because of anatomical distortion there may be difficulty in maintaining the airway if respiratory disturbance occurs during sedation. Sleep apnoea (commonly known as Pickwick syndrome) is common in overweight patients. Due to snoring at night, the patient becomes repeatedly hypoxic, and does not sleep well. This predisposes to excessive drowsiness during the day, and exaggerated responses to the sedative effects of drugs. Increasingly, these patients have continuous positive airway pressure (CPAP) devices at home to maintain their airway and breathing at night. They may need to bring these devices into hospital with them for use in the event of post-sedation respiratory difficulty, and recovery from sedation may have to occur in a high-dependency area.[5]

Allergies

Specific drug allergies should be identified and explored. For example, many patients will state that they are allergic to morphine and pethidine, but when questioned will reveal that they had in fact suffered from known side-effects such as nausea and vomiting. In such cases, reassurance can be offered and the medication used as planned. Symptoms such as rash, asthma, facial swelling or collapse may indicate a true allergy, and drugs associated with this type of reaction should be avoided. Latex allergy is becoming increasingly common, and patients with latex allergy should be nursed in a latex-free environment. This will require the procedure area to have been latex free for some hours, and no new latex-based material should be introduced into the environment during the patient's treatment.

Other factors

There are other factors which may influence whether the patient is suitable for sedation or not, particularly in the day-case (as opposed to inpatient) setting. If the patient is being allowed home on the same day as they were sedated, steps must be taken to ensure that they are discharged into a safe environment. This means that the correct social circumstances must be in place. Commonly used criteria for the discharge of day-case patients are listed in Box 3.2.

The patient must be escorted home by a responsible adult, and must be supervised at home by such an adult for at least 24 hours. There should be a phone or other method of contacting the hospital for advice if required. Patients should not be left alone to supervise themselves, or dependents such as children. If the patient is a carer for a dependent relative, arrangements such as respite care may be required. The patient should not drive, operate machinery, sign legal documents or return to work for 24 hours following the administration of sedative drugs.[6] The use of an antagonist such as flumazenil should not be assumed to allow safe discharge, as sedative symptoms may reappear later.

BOX 3.2 Typical day-case discharge criteria

Social circumstances
- The patient should be escorted home.
- The patient should be under the supervision of a responsible adult.
- The patient/responsible adult should have a means of contacting the hospital to ask for advice if complications arise.
- The patient/responsible adult must be given a written set of post-operative instructions.

Patient restrictions
For the first 24 hours following sedation it is advised that patients should not:
- drive
- operate heavy machinery
- be left unaccompanied by a responsible adult
- be left in charge of children
- return to work
- sign legal documents or make significant legal, financial or business decisions.

Summary

The sedationist has an important role in the selection of patients for sedation. With the increasing emphasis on performing procedures as day cases, it is essential that all aspects of the patient's health and social circumstances have been considered in the context of the environment and facilities within which sedation will be taking place. The responsibility for final patient risk assessment lies with the sedationist, and cannot be devolved to or assumed to lie with the referring practitioner, consultant or GP.

> **LEARNING POINTS**
>
> - The sedationist is the final link in the chain of safety which ensures that the patient is suitable for the proposed procedure and sedation in the available environment.
> - The sedationist needs to understand the common risks associated with the patient's medical conditions.
> - The sedationist needs to understand the technicalities of and complications associated with the proposed procedure or treatment.

References

1 Adams A. Epidemiology and identification of the high-risk surgical patient. In: McConachie I, editor. *Anaesthesia for the High-Risk Patient*. London: Greenwich Medical Media Ltd; 2002. pp. 1–28.

2 Janke E, Chalk V, Kinley H. *Pre-Operative Assessment. Setting a standard through learning*. Southampton: University of Southampton and the NHS Modernisation Agency; 2002.

3 Chassot P-G, Delabays A, Spahn DR. Perioperative anti-platelet therapy: the case for continuing therapy in patients at risk from myocardial infarction. *Br J Anaesth*. 2007; **99:** 316–28.

4 Watts JC, Brierley A. Midazolam for the treatment of post-operative nausea? *Anaesthesia*. 2001; **56:** 1129.

5 Association of Anaesthetists of Great Britain and Ireland. *Perioperative Management of the Morbidly Obese Patient;* www.aagbi.org/publications/guidelines/docs/Obesity07.pdf (accessed 4 August 2007).

6 Association of Anaesthetists of Great Britain and Ireland. *Day Surgery;* www.aagbi.org/publications/guidelines/docs/daysurgery05.pdf (accessed 23 January 2007).

CHAPTER 4

Principles of safety in sedation

It is vital that sedation is performed in an environment that minimises any risk to both the patient and the staff. Table 4.1 lists some of the different clinical areas outside an operating-theatre environment where sedation for procedures might reasonably be expected to occur at regular intervals. It is clear that not all of these clinical areas are exactly the same in nature, nor do they share the same personnel with the same clinical background and experience.

TABLE 4.1 Different clinical areas where sedation may regularly occur (this list is not exhaustive)

CLINICAL AREA	EXAMPLES
Radiology department	MRI scans
	CT scans
	Interventional radiology (e.g. vascular angiography)
Ward area	Painful procedures (e.g. lumbar puncture, vascular access procedures, etc.)
Emergency department	Fracture manipulation
	Dislocation manipulation
	Minor surgical procedures
Endoscopy suites	Bronchoscopy
	Gastroscopy
	Endoscopic ultrasonography
	Colonoscopy

cont.

CLINICAL AREA	EXAMPLES
Angiography suites	Angiography
	Angioplasty
	Co-ablation procedures

Some of these clinical areas may be remote from the main hospital, or even contained within a totally separate, stand-alone, isolated unit, and as such present challenges of their own.[1,2] The Royal College of Anaesthetists recently published recommendations relating to the standards expected when giving anaesthetics in 'remote sites.'[3] These suggest that anaesthetists should adhere to the same standards of practice in remote areas as they would do in a main operating theatre. In other words, the anaesthetist must ensure that they are practising as safely in isolated clinical environments as they would be able to practise in their normal workplace. It may not be practicable to equip every area where sedation is performed in the same manner as an operating theatre, but the core facilities must be similar.[4,5]

The standards of the environment required for safe sedation have not been defined as strictly as those required for anaesthesia, but several documents and societies have tried to address them appropriately. In essence, the sedation facility must adhere to standards that are akin to those for anaesthesia, but not necessarily exactly the same. Table 4.2 lists some considerations with regard to sedation facilities, gleaned from many different guidelines and reports.

Unless areas in which sedation is provided are within the main operating theatre, it is possible that they may not be fitted with dedicated equipment, or alternatively they may be equipped with devices that have previously been used in the theatres, but which have been replaced there by newer models. It is important for staff in sedation facilities which receive such devices to remember that, when in theatre, this equipment will have been subject to rigorous, sometimes daily, safety checks and services. In fact, every anaesthetist is trained to perform a minimum safety check on their machines before using them.[4] Staff in suites that are not attached to theatres which receive such decanted equipment should ensure that they are checked as regularly as is recommended, even if they are not often used. For example, in the case of older equipment it is entirely possible that spare parts would not be immediately available (or even available at all) if the devices started to malfunction. Improperly maintained equipment can fail when it is most needed (*see* Box 4.1), with disastrous consequences for the patient. It is unlikely that the Courts would look favourably on such lapses if legal action resulted.

TABLE 4.2 Aspects to be considered when ensuring that an environment is safe for sedation

CONSIDERATION	FACTORS REQUIRED
Appropriate back-up support in case of emergency	Emergency equipment and drugs
	Skilled staff in sedation area
	Oxygen supply
	Airway equipment
	Access to relevant emergency teams (e.g. 'crash team')
Appropriate staff skill base	Training in routine sedation management, including recovery
	Ability to deal with emergency situations (e.g. inappropriately deep sedation, life support skills)
Appropriate monitoring equipment available	Pulse oximeter
	Capnograph
	ECG monitor
	Blood pressure monitor
	Ability to record and act on data appropriately
Ability to preserve patient dignity and privacy	Facilities
	Staffing
	Equipment
Appropriate recovery facilities	Equipment
	Monitoring
	Staffing
	Discharge criteria

BOX 4.1 Failure to maintain equipment

An anaesthetic registrar received an emergency SOS call to an angiography suite, which was remote from the main hospital building. Taking some anaesthetic drugs with him, the registrar ran to the source of the emergency. When he arrived he found that a patient had rapidly deteriorated during an emergency percutaneous intervention, as the catheterisation had stimulated an aortic and coronary artery dissection. The patient was grey, clammy, cyanosed and sitting up on the catheter table with pulmonary oedema literally gushing from his mouth. A theatre auxiliary was trying to administer oxygen to the patient through a Venturi mask from a small portable oxygen cylinder. Two cardiology doctors were fully scrubbed, manipulating the cardiac catheter which was still *in situ*. The cardiologists shouted at the registrar to intubate the patient immediately, but the registrar insisted on checking the available emergency equipment first. During the checks he noted the following:

- The angiography suite did not have piped oxygen. The sole supply was from one small portable cylinder (currently in use by the auxiliary).
- An old Boyle's-type theatre anaesthetic machine was available. This did have oxygen cylinders attached. However, it became clear that the machine had not been serviced or checked recently as:
  - the oxygen cylinders were empty
  - the spare oxygen cylinder in the storage area was also empty
  - no breathing system was attached to the machine, or immediately available
  - if a breathing system had been available, there was no means of actually connecting it to an endotracheal tube, as all of the available connectors had been jammed together and were inseparable and unusable.
- Laryngoscopes were available, but all of the bulbs and batteries were dead.
- If he had intubated the patient, there would be no means of keeping the patient asleep, as although there was a vaporiser on the anaesthetic machine, it was empty, and there was no supply of anaesthetic vapour available in the suite. The only available anaesthetic-type drugs were diazepam and morphine.
- Apart from an electrocardiograph, no other monitoring equipment was available.

In other words, if he had succumbed to the pressure being exerted by the cardiologists, the registrar would have anaesthetised the patient, and if he had been able to intubate without a working laryngoscope, he would have been unable either to deliver oxygen to the patient, or to keep him anaesthetised and stable, or to monitor his condition. Fortunately, when he had been called, he had immediately asked the anaesthetic nurse from theatre to attend with some basic equipment. The nurse arrived some minutes later, and when the deficiencies in the available equipment had been corrected, the patient was safely anaesthetised, the procedure was completed, and the patient was then transferred to the ITU. The cardiologists attempted to complain about the anaesthetic registrar because of what they felt was an 'unacceptable delay' in anaesthetising the patient. However, the complaint was dropped rapidly when the very poor standards of the facilities that they were using were highlighted. The patient underwent corrective surgery, and survived.

Although the hospital has to ensure that all of the available equipment is serviced, checked and meets safety standards, it is the responsibility of the sedationist to ensure that the equipment and treatment area are safe to use before a procedure is started.

The considerations highlighted in this chapter apply not only to the environment in which sedation is taking place, but also to the environment in which the patient will be recovering.

Oxygen supply

As the most common dangerous complication that can arise from sedation is likely to be an airway problem resulting in hypoxia, it is recommended that patients undergoing sedation receive oxygen-supplemented air. It is also possible that a sudden deterioration in the patient's underlying condition may warrant urgent intervention, including an increase in the amount of oxygen administered, or a change in the way that it is given. The sedation environment must therefore include a reliable supply of oxygen, and various means of delivering that supply safely to the patient. Some problems that have arisen with regard to oxygen supply are described in Box 4.2.

BOX 4.2 Human errors with regard to oxygen supply

The National Patient Safety Agency (NPSA) examined a series of 200 critical incidents, 35 of which involved the administration of oxygen to patients. Many of these mistakes concerned a fundamental failure to understand how the equipment worked. Some oxygen masks were correctly attached to full cylinders, but the cylinder was not switched on. In other cases there was a delay in giving oxygen, due to slow changeover of empty cylinders. Four cases concerned the oxygen mask being connected to the wall medical air outlet rather than the wall oxygen outlet.

National Patient Safety Agency Patient Safety Bulletin, 3 April 2007.

Oxygen pipelines

In hospitals and purpose-built clinics, oxygen will be supplied either from a remote main cylinder manifold, or from a liquid oxygen tank, via pipelines, to the oxygen outlet on the wall. These pipelines will be subject to regular monitoring and maintenance by trained specialists. The sedationist and clinical staff are obviously not responsible for ensuring the integrity of the supply. However, they are responsible for ensuring that oxygen is being delivered from the pipeline to the patient, and for the management of any crisis, such as pipeline failure.[6] This means that the supply must be checked before the patient is treated, and that the patient and the supply must be adequately monitored during sedation.

A variety of alarms that warn of low oxygen pressure should be in use. Some of these are inherent in the pipeline system and warn of a failure of supply to an entire clinical area. Others will be intrinsic to devices such as modern anaesthetic machines, and will warn of a supply failure between the wall outlet and the patient. If an anaesthetic machine is being utilised, staff should ensure that oxygen failure alarms and inspired oxygen monitors are being used.

The wall outlet will allow only the correct-shaped pipeline connector from an anaesthetic machine to be inserted. This is particularly important when an area receives piped supplies of multiple gases, such as nitrous oxide or medical air.

An oxygen flow meter, rather than a pipe from an anaesthetic machine, can also be connected to these outlets. A flow meter can be connected to simple oxygen delivery devices such as face masks, or self-inflating bags.

Oxygen cylinders

Oxygen can be supplied from an anaesthetic machine, or through a flow meter, via a local gas cylinder. The gas cylinder is connected via the head to a yoke on the oxygen delivery device. Although they are clearly labelled according to standard ISO/R32, medical gas cylinders are also colour coded to prevent confusion according to BS 1319 (see Table 4.3). However, the system as detailed within the UK will soon be altered to BS EN 1089-3, standardising colours across Europe. In the latter standard, the 'shoulder' of the cylinder will remain the same colour as at present, but the medical gas companies are free to paint the body of the cylinder any colour they wish. The European Industrial Gas Association has recommended that all medical gas cylinders should have bodies that are painted white, to distinguish them from non-medical gases. This would mean, for example, that an oxygen cylinder would have a white body and a white shoulder; and a nitrous oxide cylinder would be white with a blue shoulder.[7]

In order to prevent connection to the wrong supply pipeline, the yoke (in addition to the connectors) is pin index coded. This simple system has six identified positions on the cylinder head which could contain holes. These positions overlap, so that a cylinder head could not, for example, have holes drilled in position 1 and position 2, or position 5 and 6. These holes will correspond with the position of pins on the anaesthetic machine or flow meter yoke. The pin positions are unique to each gas, and should therefore prevent a cylinder from being connected to an incorrect yoke.

TABLE 4.3 Current colour coding of medical gas cylinders in the UK

GAS	CYLINDER BODY COLOUR	CYLINDER SHOULDER COLOUR
Oxygen	Black	White
Nitrous oxide	Blue	Blue
Entonox	Blue	Blue and white
Air	Grey	White and black
Carbon dioxide	Grey	Grey

Cylinders come in a variety of sizes, containing different volumes of gases. It is important to remember that the contents of cylinders are pressurised, and that the pressure inside the cylinder is read through an appropriate gauge. In the case of oxygen, the lower the pressure reading on the valve, the lower the amount of oxygen in the cylinder, because oxygen is stored entirely in the gaseous state in the cylinder. However, in the case of nitrous oxide and Entonox, the gas is stored inside the cylinder over a liquid phase. The liquid evaporates, replenishing the gas phase as it is used. Therefore the pressure gauge reading will not start to fall until the liquid phase has been completely used up, at which point the remaining gas will be rapidly exhausted.

BOX 4.3 Failure to supply oxygen appropriately

A 55-year-old woman died during general anaesthesia for an ENT procedure. Instead of a ventilator, the endotracheal tube had been connected directly to an oxygen cylinder. When the oxygen supply was turned on, the woman received over 1000 litres of oxygen within a few minutes, inflating 'to resemble a *Michelin Man* of the tyre advertisements.' The locum anaesthetist supervising the woman's management was convicted of manslaughter, and was sentenced to 6 months' imprisonment.

Anaesthetist convicted of manslaughter. *Guardian*, 31 July 1990.

Sedationists who use devices which incorporate a cylinder supply of oxygen should ensure that they are familiar with all aspects of oxygen supply, particularly what action they should take in the event of a failure. This means that they need to understand all of the aspects outlined above, and should possess skills such as the ability to replace an empty cylinder.

Oxygen is supplied from cylinders and pipelines at high pressure, and should pass through an appropriate pressure-reducing device before being supplied to a patient (*see* Box 4.3).

Oxygen flow meters

Flow meters are usually an intrinsic component of an anaesthetic machine, a gas cylinder or a pipeline yoke. They normally consist of a bobbin within a calibrated transparent tube. When the oxygen supply is turned on, the bobbin should rise to a level that indicates the gas flow being supplied. The bobbin should be seen to be spinning, to ensure that it is not stuck. The physics relating to such a seemingly simple device are quite complex, and do not need to be described in detail here. The flow meter may be inaccurate if it is not positioned vertically.

Oxygen delivery systems

Broadly speaking, oxygen delivery systems can be divided into two types, namely *closed/semi-closed* and *open*. Closed and semi-closed systems should basically be considered as anaesthetic breathing circuits. Different types of circuits have different functioning characteristics. For example, the rate of gas flow through the breathing system necessary to prevent the patient re-breathing their own exhaled carbon dioxide can vary markedly. These systems should generally only be utilised by those trained in their use. However, in an emergency situation, if such a system is being used, the oxygen flow rate should be as high as possible.

Open oxygen delivery systems include nasal cannulae and oxygen face masks. In these systems the term 'open' implies that the oxygen flow has the potential to be diluted by room air, which means that the concentration of oxygen delivered can vary widely. Again, different systems are available, and they have different functioning characteristics. Broadly speaking there are two types of open oxygen delivery system, characterised by whether the oxygen concentration that the patient breathes in is *variable* or *fixed*.

Variable-performance open oxygen delivery systems

With variable-performance systems, the oxygen delivery to the patient varies with the gas flow that is set, and with the patient's breathing pattern.

In general, as the oxygen flow increases, the fractional inspired oxygen concentration increases. However, as the respiratory rate increases, the inspired oxygen concentration tends to decrease because of re-breathing and air entrainment.[8]

Nasal cannulae

These consist of simple tubes that are placed in the patient's nostrils. Oxygen flow is usually limited to 4 litres per minute maximum in order to minimise discomfort and drying of mucous membranes. Nasal cannulae can reliably deliver up to 30% oxygen if used in this manner. New systems are available that will allow warming and humidification of oxygen delivered by nasal cannulae, thereby increasing the rate of gas flow that can be tolerated.

Oxygen face masks

Variable-concentration oxygen delivery masks are often referred to as Hudson-type masks, and are commonly used in the ward situation, fitting loosely over the nose and mouth. An inspired oxygen concentration of up to 50% can be achieved in most circumstances when oxygen flow rates are set at 6–10 litres/minute (*see* Table 4.4). An oxygen flow rate of 5 litres/minute or below will not be high enough to prevent the re-breathing of exhaled gas.

TABLE 4.4 Variable oxygen delivery mask performance[8]

VARIABLE OXYGEN DELIVERY DEVICE	OXYGEN FLOW RATE (L/MIN)	RESULTANT OXYGEN CONCENTRATION (%)
Nasal cannulae	1	24
	2	28
	4	36
Hudson-type mask	5–6	40
	9–10	60
Hudson-type non re-breather	10–12	80–100

The oxygen delivery of variable-concentration masks can be increased by attaching a reservoir bag. The bag fills with oxygen, and reduces the likelihood of re-breathing, as well as increasing the inspired oxygen concentration to over 80%. These masks are commonly used in emergency departments and ambulances. The gas flow should be adjusted so that the reservoir bag does not deflate by more than a third during inspiration.

Fixed-performance open oxygen delivery systems

Fixed-concentration masks are designed to deliver a set inspired concentration of oxygen over a range of oxygen flow rates, irrespective of the patient's pattern of breathing. They are commonly referred to as 'Venturi masks.' The masks are usually labelled to indicate what concentration of oxygen they will deliver, as well as being colour coded.[9] Table 4.5 summarises the characteristics of these devices.

TABLE 4.5 Fixed oxygen delivery mask colour coding[9]

VALVE COLOUR	OXYGEN FLOW RATE (L/MIN)	RESULTANT OXYGEN CONCENTRATION DELIVERED (%)
Blue	2	24
White	4	28
Yellow	6	35
Red	8	40
Green	12	60

Anaesthetic machine

This is commonly referred to as the 'Boyle's machine', after the anaesthetist credited with its invention in 1917.[10,11] Essentially an anaesthetic machine consists of a mobile framework of pipes through which an oxygen supply (from either pipelines or cylinders) can be delivered to the patient. The machine has a flow meter through which the flow of oxygen (usually measured in litres/minute) and the mixture of gases (usually expressed as fractional inspired oxygen concentration, or FiO_2 %) can be adjusted. The machine contains valves that will reduce the high-pressure gas flow received into a low-pressure flow in order to avoid injury to the patient. There is also a facility to allow oxygen to be supplied directly to the patient, bypassing much of the machine, in the event of an emergency. In addition, the machine receives a supply of other gases (nitrous oxide or air), which also arrives from mounted cylinders or pipelines via pressure-reducing devices. These are also adjustable via the flow meter. The machine must *not* allow a hypoxic gas mixture to be delivered, and therefore should have several safety features. These include oxygen failure alarms, colour-coded flow-meter knobs, a standard flow-meter set-up, and an inability to turn the oxygen off completely – or, similarly, an inability to turn on nitrous oxide without oxygen also being supplied at a non-hypoxic concentration. This is referred to as the *anti-hypoxic mixture protection*.

The Association of Anaesthetists of Great Britain and Ireland (AAGBI) has produced a checklist that every user of such a machine should ensure has been completed before the machine can be used.[4] This is summarised in Table 4.6. However, every healthcare worker who is using such a device must ensure that they are intimately familiar with it. Although each machine is based upon the same basic layout, there can be considerable variation in construction and function. For example, older machines might allow a cylinder of carbon dioxide gas to be attached, or might not have anti-hypoxic mixture protection. Failure to appreciate this can lead to clinical catastrophes in unskilled hands (for examples of such clinical scenarios, *see* Boxes 4.4 and 4.5).

TABLE 4.6 Abbreviated anaesthetic machine checklist[4]

Check that the machine is plugged in and switched on (if appropriate).
Check that all monitoring devices (especially capnograph, pulse oximeter and oxygen analyser) are working, and that sampling lines are not obstructed.
Check that each gas pipeline is correctly inserted into the correct outlet on the wall. Ensure that adequate oxygen is available in the back-up machine-mounted cylinder. Use the oxygen analyser to ensure that the machine is receiving and dispensing oxygen. Ensure that non-used cylinder spaces are blanked off. Ensure that pipeline pressure readings do not exceed 400–500 kPa.
Check that the flow meter is working correctly. Ensure that the bobbin rises and rotates. Ensure that the anti-hypoxia mixture device works, and that the emergency oxygen bypass works.
Ensure that the vaporisers are filled and mounted correctly, and that there are no gas leaks when they are switched on.
Check that the breathing system is fitted correctly, that it is not obstructed, and that when it is occluded, pressure-release alarms work correctly.
Check that the ventilator is functioning and connected appropriately.
Check that the necessary ancillary equipment is available and functioning.
Ensure that there is an alternative means of ventilating the patient in the event of machine failure.

BOX 4.4 Failure to use equipment properly

N, a 3-year-old girl, collapsed and suffered convulsions after receiving a flu jab at her general practitioner's surgery. She was taken to the local Accident and Emergency department, where the consultant in charge, Dr H, decided to give her high-flow oxygen from an anaesthetic machine that was kept in the department for emergencies. Unfortunately, in the heat of the moment,

Dr H inadvertently turned on the nitrous oxide valve rather than the oxygen valve. As it was an old machine, discarded by theatres, it did not have an anti-hypoxic mixture guard, and N received 100% nitrous oxide. It was not realised that she was not receiving oxygen for nearly 10 minutes, by which time she had suffered fatal brain damage. Initially a manslaughter charge was considered, but an inquest concluded that Dr H had made a genuine mistake. He underwent re-training. As a result of this error, the Chief Medical Officer ordered that all anaesthetic machines in current use should be fitted with a hypoxic mixture alarm.

Fatal mix-up doctor can work again. BBC News, 22 March 2001; http://news.bbc.co.uk/1/hi/health/1235745.stm (accessed 15 April 2007)

Doctor sobs over hospital blunder. BBC News, 12 April 2002; http://news.bbc.co.uk/1/hi/england/1925267.stm (accessed 15 April 2007)

BOX 4.5 Failure to check machine, leading to hypoxia

A boy died during dental surgery at a dental practice. He had been given nitrous oxide instead of oxygen because the tubing was wrongly connected, and the anaesthetist failed to check the equipment. The child's underlying health problems made resuscitation more difficult, but no one present had obtained his medical history. The judge recorded that 'This offence was one of the most gross negligence.' The anaesthetist was sentenced to 6 months' imprisonment.

Anaesthetist jailed over death. *Daily Telegraph*, 30 July 1999.

Specific anaesthetic gas machines have been designed for use in dental practice. These 'relative analgesia' machines deliver a mixture of oxygen and nitrous oxide through a non-re-breathing circuit. They share some of the safety features and functions of anaesthetic machines, and can be used to deliver anaesthetic vapours. Whatever type of machine is available, if it is to be used, the sedationist will need to ensure that it has been checked before commencing.

Airway support devices

If the respiration of a patient is insufficient, the sedationist will need to support ventilation to prevent hypoxia. It is therefore recommended that the sedationist should be skilled in the use of self-inflating bags, face masks and assorted airway equipment in order to relieve this problem. The most essential skill is to realise when such devices may be required, and to decide which is the most appropriate device to use in a particular situation.

Self-inflating bag

This apparatus consists of a bag that re-inflates after squeezing. This is attached at one end to a one-way flow valve that can be connected to a face mask or other apparatus, while at the other end it should also have the facility for receiving supplementary oxygen. Once the airway is patent and the face mask is held on the face, this apparatus can be used to hand ventilate the patient. The efficiency of the self-inflating bag is highly dependent upon the skill and technique of the user.

Airway adjuncts

Oropharyngeal airways (commonly known as 'Guedel airways') come in a variety of sizes. They are designed to slide into the mouth and sit over the back of the tongue, creating a clear passage for suction or oxygenation from the atmosphere to the pharynx. If the patient can tolerate the insertion of such an airway, this means that they have no working airway reflexes – a state that is indicative of anaesthesia or unconsciousness. *Nasopharyngeal airways* are similar, but are designed to slide into the nostril to the back of the pharynx. Unskilled insertion is associated with nasal bleeding. The ability to use such devices is essential in the rescue of patients with breathing problems secondary to over-sedation.

Laryngeal mask airway (LMA)

The LMA consists of an oval-shaped inflatable cuff attached to a curved tube. It is designed to be inserted blindly into the mouth and to sit in the pharynx over the larynx. This can secure an effective airway in an anaesthetised or collapsed patient, but does not protect the airway from aspiration events. It has been shown that minimal training can result in effective insertion by trainees in over 90% of situations. The tube of the mask can be attached to a breathing system to allow either spontaneous or hand/mechanical ventilation. Anaesthetists provide training in the use of such devices for paramedics and others in the theatre environment. It is recommended that the sedationist is familiar with the use and limitations of this device, which can be of great assistance if the patient develops breathing difficulties.

Endotracheal (ET) tubes

ET tubes are designed to be inserted through the larynx into the trachea when the patient is anaesthetised or collapsed. They secure the airway and prevent aspiration. A certain degree of skill is required to place them properly, so it is unlikely that a non-anaesthetic sedationist would be expected to intubate in the event of an emergency.

Laryngoscopes

A laryngoscope is designed to enable visualisation of the larynx. It consists of a blade, containing a light source, which is inserted into the mouth, and is attached to a handle. It is used to aid the insertion of an ET tube during anaesthesia.

Other airway devices

Other airway devices are available but, at the time of writing, few of them have been properly assessed either in emergency situations or in unskilled hands. It is assumed that the sedationist will know what equipment their organisation has readily available for them to use in an emergency, and how to utilise it correctly.

Other essential equipment

Defibrillators

The usual cardiac rhythms associated with sudden cardiac arrest in adults are ventricular fibrillation (VF) and pulseless ventricular tachycardia (VT). Both of these cardiac arrhythmias are treated by administering a defibrillatory shock. In simple terms, an electrical discharge is administered to provide a global shock to the heart, in order to resynchronise electrical pacemaker activity. Occasionally, defibrillators can be used to treat other cardiac disturbances. Many different types of defibrillator exist, and it is important that those intending to use them in an emergency can do so properly and safely. Modern defibrillators may work on a totally automatic basis, or can issue instructions to a manual operator. However, training in their use is still essential, as unskilled usage can result in harm to both patient and staff. It is suggested that staff attend either a nationally recognised resuscitation course, or local training, at regular intervals.

Infusion devices

Increased interest in the use of propofol for sedation, particularly in target-controlled infusions (*see* Chapter 5), means that the sedationist will need to understand the uses and limitations of infusion devices. The British Medicines and Healthcare Regulatory Agency has stated its concern about the large number of critical incidents that are associated with such devices, most of which are attributable to human error. This is particularly alarming in view of the fact that such devices are ubiquitous throughout a modern hospital. Problems occur because of incorrect pump selection, incorrect programming, incorrect syringe selection, or problems with giving sets, valves and connectors.

Syringe-driver pumps appear deceptively simple – the drug is loaded into a syringe, and the syringe is placed inside the driver. The driver then compresses the syringe plunger at a set rate, delivering the drug to the patient over a set time period. Unfortunately, many of these drivers alter the rate of delivery depending upon syringe characteristics, so the machine needs to be programmed with the correct *make* of syringe, otherwise the driving pressure, and therefore the rate of drug delivery, will be incorrect. The internal diameter of the giving set attached to the syringe may also cause inaccuracy if it is not the type recommended by the manufacturer. In addition, many syringe drivers are designed to be multipurpose, in that they can be programmed to deliver the drug on the basis of ml/hour, ml/minute, mg/kg or mcg/kg/minute, and the sedationist must ensure that they have selected the correct programme. Drug errors are common when the medication placed inside the syringe has to be drawn up manually and/ or diluted by hand. It is far better for such drug solutions to be prepared in advance, if possible, by the pharmacy department. Propofol is already available in pre-packaged syringes, but even then errors can occur, as it is available in both 1% and 2% solutions.

The position of the pump relative to the patient can also cause errors. If the pump is more than 100 cm above the patient, there is a possibility that gravity may overcome the syringe barrel resistance, leading to excess dosage. If the connector is not secure, or there is a crack in the closed system that allows air to enter it, the contents of the syringe may siphon into the patient. The use of anti-siphon valves as part of the giving set is recommended. Sometimes other fluids (e.g. antibiotics, saline, etc.) are also attached to the same cannula to which the sedation giving set is attached, in which case anti-reflux valves, which prevent the backtracking of the drug into the supplementary fluid, should be used.[12] Deaths have been reported when multiple infusions through different sites in the same patient have been used, because the wrong drug has been connected to the wrong drip.[13]

Monitoring

The term 'monitoring' is often used to refer exclusively to the electronic technology attached to the patient in order to measure various physiological parameters. In reality, 'monitoring' encompasses a much broader concept than this. It is a defined link between the patient's physiology (and how it reacts to an intervention) and the observer who is utilising the measuring devices. If this concept is elaborated upon, it is clear that monitoring is a *process* and that it serves the function of alerting the observer to the maintenance of, or changes in, the patient's current condition. It also follows that the modes of monitoring which are utilised will depend upon the observer's perception of what monitors are appropriate, according to the positive or adverse effects that are likely to occur in response to an intervention. In addition, it follows that the efficiency of the monitoring process will depend upon the type of monitor used, its ability to function, and the ability of the observer to understand and act upon the information that the monitor provides. There are therefore several stages in this framework at which the monitoring process can fail.

The use of 'monitoring' in itself does not ensure the safety of the patient.[14] There is no point in utilising a monitor to observe the patient's condition if the monitor itself is not being watched or understood (*see* Boxes 4.6 and 4.7). Equally, if the observer is unable to interpret the data that are produced, the monitoring process will become irrelevant. For example, if a high blood sugar level is measured, this information should trigger a response in the observer other than merely recording that fact – whether this is to repeat the test, inform someone else, obtain assistance or treat the patient. In other words, a monitor is useless if the observer cannot understand and interpret what it is telling them, and then decide upon appropriate action. This sounds like common sense, but it is failures such as this that have led to cases where staff have faithfully recorded a patient's preventable decline, without realising that intervention was necessary. Such circumstances have led to the introduction of so-called 'early warning scores' (EWS) on wards. These systems assign a numerical value to normally recorded ward patient observations (respiratory rate, heart rate, blood pressure, body temperature, level of consciousness, etc.). Once the observations have been recorded, the scores are totalled. If the total score is greater than a pre-set trigger value, the observer should ensure that someone is informed and that action is taken. Some of these charts are even colour coded to reinforce the recognition of danger signs.

BOX 4.6 The importance of understanding the monitoring system

A final-year student nurse was given the task of observing a patient who had just been transferred to theatre recovery following a hip replacement operation. A short time later the recovery emergency alarm sounded. When the anaesthetist arrived, the student nurse explained that the patient had 'gone into asystole' according to the ECG monitor trace. Fortunately, the patient was still fully conscious and comfortable, and wanted to know 'what all the fuss was about.' The patient had not in fact arrested. The ECG leads had become disconnected, and the nurse had triggered the alarm on the basis of the faulty trace, without first checking the patient.

BOX 4.7 Failure to observe the monitoring

An anaesthetist, Dr B, was referred to a GMC Fitness to Practise panel due to failure to maintain appropriate vigilance during a series of operations. On one occasion he had allegedly fallen asleep during the operation, and on another it was alleged that, after the operation had started, he watched a feature film DVD on a laptop computer while wearing headphones. He was suspended from the medical register for one month and underwent re-training.

Dayani A. Revealed: the sleep op doc. *Birmingham Mail*, 28 July 2005.
Dayani A. 'Snoozing' doc returns to work. *Birmingham Mail*, 3 August 2006.

The standards for the monitoring of patients undergoing *anaesthesia* have been established by the Association of Anaesthetists since 1994, and are currently in their fourth edition.[5] They suggest that so-called 'minimum monitoring' should consist of pulse oximetry, non-invasive blood pressure (NIBP) monitoring, capnometry and an electrocardiograph (ECG), and also that 'the same standards of monitoring apply when the anaesthetist is responsible for a local/regional anaesthetic or sedative technique for an operative procedure', irrespective of duration or location. However, they do not fully define what is meant by an 'operative procedure.' For example, a colonoscopy is regarded by many as an investigation rather than an operation.

As mentioned previously, in sedation the patient should remain conscious but calm, and it could be argued that the monitoring standards described above can be relaxed in many circumstances. For example, it may be possible to monitor a patient who is undergoing a minor procedure safely with only a pulse oximeter. However, this is a judgement that can only be made when the sedationist has thoroughly considered all of the issues relating to the patient. The level of monitoring required will depend upon several factors, including the following:

➺ **Patient-related factors:** A patient who has an underlying disease may require specific monitoring as standard. For example, a patient with a pacemaker or an implantable cardiac defibrillator may always require ECG monitoring. A patient with diabetes may need to have their blood sugar level checked pre-, peri- and post-operatively. A patient with obstructive sleep apnoea may require capnography.

➺ **Procedure-related factors:** Certain procedures may be commonly expected to precipitate a certain physiological response (e.g. bradycardia), and this may dictate the level of monitoring required.

However, it is also important to take into account practicalities. For example, a patient who is undergoing a cataract operation may not be able to keep as still as required if repeated use of an automatic blood pressure cuff becomes distracting.

In general, however, it is recommended that the minimum standards set out by the AAGBI are considered for all patients undergoing sedation. If these standards are to be varied by an organisation for a particular group of patients, this should be a policy decision made after proper consideration and consultation by appropriate personnel. Even then the sedationist would have to consider which patient, or groups of patients, may require more or less monitoring than this standard on some occasions. However, it is important to remember that if a complication occurs, the sedationist will be expected to justify any decision that they made to change the level of available monitoring.

It is good practice for the sedationist to ensure that the parameters which they have gone to the trouble of monitoring are documented properly. As a general rule, it is expected that the data will be recorded at 5-minute intervals on a time-based chart, relating the recorded events chronologically to any interventions (drugs given, etc.). Some monitors can also record and print data, but this does not release the sedationist from the responsibility of observing the monitors and ensuring that the results are collated.

One of the most useful functions of monitors is their ability to alert the observer to a measured abnormality by the use of alarm systems. Many monitors have a 'default' alarm setting (e.g. an alarm sounding if the heart rate falls below 60 beats/minute) set by the manufacturer, which has been judged to be suitable for the majority of patients. However, there is a facility to vary the alarm settings if necessary for an individual patient (e.g. alarm sounding if the heart rate falls below 50 beats/minute). This will avoid spurious alerts by the machine to readings that are in fact 'normal' for a particular individual. The sedationist should assess what alarm limits will be required, and whether they should be varied.

When an alarm sounds, the observer must then decide whether or not the highlighted abnormality requires intervention of some kind. This decision should be based upon observation of the patient's condition compared with their pre-operative state, and a rigorous check of the equipment. There is a facility to silence an alarm for a short period if it is interfering with concentration. However, an alarm that is sounding should never be ignored or treated lightly, and the alarm system itself should never be switched off or disabled completely.

It follows therefore that in order to interpret and act upon information supplied by the monitor that is being utilised, the sedationist needs to have a complete understanding of how the monitor works, what it measures, and what its limitations are.

What physiological parameters should be monitored?

The physiological parameters that are measured during general anaesthesia consist of pulse rate and regularity, blood pressure, ECG, pulse oximetry and capnometry (measurement of expired carbon dioxide (CO_2) levels). Depending on the type of surgery employed, other parameters may also be monitored, such as degree of muscle relaxation, blood sugar level and body temperature. In addition, there will be monitoring of anaesthetic equipment function (ventilator alarms, syringe drivers), levels of anaesthetic agents being inhaled, levels of oxygen being inhaled, and fluid input and losses. Finally, there are also brain activity monitors, to ensure that the patient is anaesthetised.

Referring back to the definition of sedation that was presented in Chapter 1, it is clear that it may be impossible to utilise some of these monitors in some circumstances, and that it may be necessary to monitor additional parameters in others. In addition, it is likely that patients who are undergoing sedation will be having shorter procedures performed than those who are undergoing anaesthesia, and so it may be impractical to use monitoring equipment that takes a long time to set up.

In order to outline which monitoring equipment is necessary, it is essential to determine what parameters should be recorded and observed. Careful monitoring of the patient will need to continue into the recovery period.[15]

Respiratory parameters

Respiratory rate

This can be monitored either visually by the sedationist, or by means of a capnograph.

A capnograph is a device that is used to measure expired CO_2 levels – a monitoring method that is familiar to anaesthetists, but perhaps not widely used in other environments.

Gases consisting of more than one atom, such as CO_2, will absorb infra-red radiation, and a capnograph works on this principle to determine CO_2 levels in a gas mixture. Exhaled gas is sampled, subjected to infra-red light, and the amount of absorption that occurs is used to determine how much CO_2 is present. This is generally displayed on a monitor screen in two ways – as a figure (which can be expressed in mmHg, kPa or as a percentage of gas expired) and as a waveform. The waveform will give evidence of respiratory rate and regularity.

Depending on the type of device, either the exhaled gas is analysed while it is still in the main gas flow, or a small sample is diverted up a side-stream pipe into the sampling chamber. The former apparatus has a bulkier connector, designed to attach to breathing circuits. The latter type has a smaller connector which can easily be adapted for use in sedation if the connector is secured near the patient's nostril or mouth. Although the level of CO_2 displayed may not necessarily be accurate, this method can in fact effectively measure respiratory rate and pattern. Research has been done which demonstrates the usefulness of capnography in paediatric practice.[16]

Interpretation of the capnograph trace does require some training. However, an abnormally slow respiratory rate could be a sign of imminent respiratory arrest, whereas a fast respiratory rate could indicate agitation, pain, or respiratory or circulatory insufficiency.

Oxygen saturation

This is measured using a pulse oximeter.

The pulse oximeter also works on the principle of infra-red absorption. In simple terms, haemoglobin can be thought of as existing in two states – oxygenated and deoxygenated. These two states absorb different wave-lengths of red light to differing extents. By passing red light at a wavelength of 660 nm and infra-red at a wavelength of 940 nm through some tissue, and comparing how much of each wavelength has been absorbed, a ratio of oxygenated to deoxygenated haemoglobin can be calculated. The light is generated by a diode which rapidly switches on and off ('pulsing') many times per second. This allows the device to detect the difference between the pulsatile (arteriolar) and non-pulsatile (tissue capillary and venous) components of absorption.

The device gives a reading as a percentage of haemoglobin saturated with oxygen. In normal individuals breathing air, this would be expected to be in the high 90s. It is important to remember that a saturation reading of less than 90% indicates very severe hypoxia. For this reason, it is recommended that the alarms are not set below this figure.

It may be preferable to utilise an oximeter which also displays a waveform. The waveform displayed will vary with the patient's pulse rate, and can indicate the presence of arrhythmias.

In practice, use of the monitor requires a small probe to be placed on a patient's extremity (e.g. nose, ear lobe, finger, toe).

The device is very versatile, but has several important limitations. Abnormal pigments in the blood can alter light absorption characteristics. For example, a large percentage of carboxyhaemoglobin in the blood (as a result of smoke inhalation from a house fire) could cause the oximeter to persistently over-read in the presence of hypoxia. Methaemoglobin (which can result from the use of methylene blue dye) will cause the device to under-read. Jaundice may also alter readings. The device can only be accurate if the periphery that is being measured is well perfused with blood, so in the presence of circulatory shock the oximeter may not work at all. The device is often inaccurate at low levels of oxygenation. The presence of dirt or nail varnish on the hands, extraneous background light contamination or hypo-thermia can all affect the readings displayed.

ECG

It has been known for many years that the electrical activity of the heart can be displayed on an oscilloscope, and that the waveform displayed has a typical configuration. The use of ECGs not only allows monitoring of rate and rhythm, but can also indicate the presence of cardiac ischaemia.

The device is vulnerable to both electromagnetic interference (from other electrical equipment) and mechanical interference (from patient movement). In addition, because the electrical pattern displayed on the monitor depends upon the position of the leads relative to the heart, the electrodes must be placed on the patient in a standard manner, otherwise the displayed pattern could be interpreted erroneously. In most clinical operative circumstances, a three-lead display is used. The leads are colour coded such that the red lead is attached to the right shoulder, the yellow lead to the left shoulder, and the green lead to the left upper abdomen (also described by the mnemonic '**R**ight **R**ed, **L**eft ye**LL**ow, **Green** for **Spleen**').

Blood pressure

The most widely used method of measuring blood pressure is the sphygmomanometer, commonly known as the 'BP cuff.' In simple terms, a pneumatic inflatable cuff (which is attached to a manometer) is wrapped around the upper arm and inflated to above the patient's expected systolic blood pressure. If the brachial pulse is auscultated while the cuff is deflating, the observer will hear a pulse beat appear. The manometer reading at this point is taken as the systolic pressure. As deflation continues, the pulse beat will quieten and then disappear. Depending on the method utilised, either of these latter sounds can be taken as the diastolic pressure. This method relies heavily upon interpreter bias and ability.

A variety of automatic sphygmomanometers exist. In some cases, the device over- or under-reads on the first attempt, and some manufacturers recommend that several readings are taken initially to ensure accuracy. A timer on the device can be set to enable the machine to measure the blood pressure at pre-set intervals, and the device has a memory to allow past readings to be displayed. Cardiac arrhythmias and poor peripheral perfusion can render the readings inaccurate, as can an inappropriately sized cuff.

Level of consciousness

As the difference between sedation and anaesthesia is essentially determined by whether the patient can still respond to a verbal stimulus or not, it is good practice to monitor the level of consciousness of the patient. Although a variety of devices are marketed for monitoring the depth of *anaesthesia*, these are not thought to be useful for monitoring the level of sedation achieved. It is therefore simpler to use an established scoring system, such as AVPU. This simple scale requires the observer to decide whether the patient is fully **A**lert, responsive to **V**erbal stimulation (such as being asked whether they are comfortable), responsive only to **P**ainful stimulation, or **U**nresponsive. This information can then be easily recorded on the sedation record chart.

Electrical safety

Accidents caused by electricity can occur in any environment, but are a particular risk when patients are attached to electrical apparatus. Electrical wiring must be fully insulated, and electrical equipment should be properly constructed so as to avoid 'short circuits' which could 'earth' electrical current through the patient. Electrocution occurs when the current passes through a patient, causing harm and/or death. Cardiac arrhythmias and burns are common consequences of such accidents. Contraction of muscles can also occur, leading to respiratory arrest. However, the amount of current required to cause serious harm can vary depending upon current density. For example, a small-voltage current delivered accidentally via a central venous catheter to the heart can induce a fatal arrhythmia. This phenomenon is referred to as 'microshock.' Electrical discharge may also ignite flammable materials, or cause an explosion.

Electrical equipment can be categorised within one of the following three classes.

➥ **Class 1:** All accessible parts are connected to the earth. If a short circuit occurs, protective fuses ensure that the live supply to the device is stopped.

➥ **Class 2:** All accessible components are protected by two layers of non-conducting insulation, to ensure that there is no possibility of a person touching a conducting part.

➥ **Class 3:** These are devices which do not normally employ normal-voltage current, so the risk of electric shock is reduced. However, the risk of microshock may still be present.

Equipment can be further classified as type B or BF (which may allow a certain level of leakage) and type CF (which may still allow current leakage, but of a much smaller level). Only type CF equipment, such as ECG leads, is suitable for (indirect) connection to the heart.

Diathermy is often used by surgeons to cut or coagulate tissue. A high-frequency electrical current is used to create heat. In monopolar systems the current is passed between a live electrode and a neutral electrode situated some distance apart on the patient, whereas in bipolar diathermy the current is passed between the points of a forceps. Accidents have been caused by unintentional activation, or by the ignition of drapes or alcohol-based skin cleansing solutions. Diathermy may have adverse effects on pacemakers and implantable cardiac defibrillators.

There has been debate as to whether the electrical fields produced by mobile phones could interfere with monitoring devices. The current position is that this is unlikely to occur with modern equipment.[17]

Other emergency considerations

Some emergency situations arise rarely, but need to be dealt with swiftly. Life-threatening *anaphylaxis* can occur in any situation, so the sedationist should have access to all of the medication and equipment necessary to treat such an event, including nebulisers, adrenaline (epinephrine), salbutamol, etc.[18] Identification of possible avoidable allergens should be part of the patient's recorded medical history. However, patients who are allergic to one medication may well be allergic to others which have not yet been identified. Antibiotics are a common precipitant, but patients may be allergic to substances such as latex in the operator's gloves. If a patient is known to be allergic to latex, the theatre will have to be specially prepared. This should include removal of all latex-containing equipment from the treatment area. Features of anaphylaxis include the development of a rash, bronchospasm, swelling and hypotension. Even if treated, cardiovascular collapse may result. Initial treatment of a severe anaphylactic reaction is summarised in Table 4.7. Some of these treatments will need to occur simultaneously, depending on the symptoms manifested by the patient. The doses quoted are for adults. Blood tests to confirm anaphylaxis, such as serum tryptase, will need to be performed.

TABLE 4.7 Summary of treatment of a severe anaphylactic reaction during sedation

Call for assistance
Stop (or reduce as much as possible) exposure to any possible cause.
Stop the investigation/procedure as soon as possible.
Administer 100% oxygen. Support the airway if necessary. Treat bronchospasm with nebulised salbutamol.
Support the blood pressure by administering fluid.
Administer adrenaline intramuscularly, 0.5–1 mg. Repeat as indicated every 10 minutes.
Administer intravenous antihistamine (e.g. chlorpheniramine, 10 mg).
Later treatment should include administration of steroids, referral to intensive care, and follow-up investigation.

Local anaesthetic toxicity is rare, but can result from either an overdose, or inadvertent administration of local anaesthetic into a blood vessel. Patients who have received an intravenous injection will complain of a variety of symptoms, including a metallic taste and periorbital numbness. They may become agitated and hypotensive. Respiratory and cardiac arrest can occur, and may even be the first symptom. This can result in a refractory ventricular fibrillation. Current opinion is that this event may be treated by the administration of intralipid solutions as well as other normal supportive measures. Areas where sedation is used in conjunction with local anaesthesia should have access to such solutions. A suggested regime is 1.5 mg/kg over 30 to 60 minutes intravenously on recognition of a local anaesthetic toxicity reaction, or on recognition of overdose, followed by repeated boluses of 1 mg/kg if symptoms persist.[19–21]

Resuscitation skills

All staff should be aware of the actions to take in an emergency, including appropriate resuscitation measures. Where sedation is taking place in a suite that is part of a well-provisioned hospital with cardiac arrest team support, it may be that basic life support skills (i.e. the ability to recognise that a cardiac arrest has occurred, support the airway and initiate cardiopulmonary resuscitation, or CPR) are the only resuscitation skills required by staff. However, where sedation is being administered in a remote site it might be decided that more advanced skills should be immediately available. Formal training on an Acute Cardiac Life Support (ACLS) course or a locally validated similar event may be equally acceptable. However, it is important that these skills are updated at regular intervals, particularly as the guidelines as to what constitutes best practice change as the evidence base develops. A summary of the current resuscitation guideline is shown in Table 4.8. Updated versions of these procedures will be available from the Resuscitation Council (UK) (www.resus.org.uk/SiteIndx.htm) or other similar national bodies. Staff should have the opportunity to regularly practise common emergency scenarios.

TABLE 4.8 Summary of adult CPR guidelines

Assess the level of consciousness, Airway, Breathing and Circulation.
Summon assistance.
Stop the investigation/treatment.
Open the airway. Administer oxygen via mouth-to-mouth respiration, or via a self-inflating bag and face mask.
If the patient has no pulse, commence chest compressions in a ratio of 30 compressions to 2 breaths.
Ensure that the patient is attached to a cardiac monitor, and analyse the rhythm.
If the patient has no pulse, and is in ventricular fibrillation or ventricular tachycardia, defibrillate according to the current guideline.
If the patient has no pulse and is in asystole or showing signs of electrical cardiac activity, continue CPR.
Administer 1 mg of adrenaline every 3 minutes.
Look for and treat possible causes (e.g. pneumothorax, cardiac tamponade, drug toxicity, pulmonary embolus, hypoxia, hypovolaemia, etc.).

Critical incidents[22]

A critical incident is an event which causes actual harm, or which has the potential to cause harm, to a patient or staff. It is essential that such incidents are logged and recorded, so that a root cause analysis can be performed, and any lessons that need to be learned can be identified and disseminated.

Such an event, even if not fatal, can be a traumatic experience for all staff involved. This can be particularly stressful if an event occurs in an outlying clinic or a private facility, as staff will feel vulnerable and isolated, and may not be able to access the normal supportive structures available in the NHS.

When a catastrophe occurs, staff should make the care and treatment of the patient their immediate concern. This duty will extend after death, and includes informing and supporting the relatives, and adhering to appropriate legal and religious procedures where appropriate.

Those involved should make detailed notes, which should be as contemporaneous as possible. They should be dated, timed and signed. During resuscitation, one team member should be allocated to the recording of treatments and times if possible. Otherwise this should occur as soon as is practicable afterwards. Individuals may need to keep copies of the notes and their statements, but should ensure that confidentiality is maintained.

Discussions with relatives should be open and honest. Saying 'sorry' does not amount to accepting liability. The coroner should be informed. Lines and tubes should be left *in situ* in the body, or if they are removed, careful note should be made of their location. There should be a 'debriefing' for all of the staff involved, so that any concerns about events can be aired and examined in a neutral, non-threatening atmosphere.

Organisations should have procedures in place for dealing with tragic circumstances such as these, including how to deal with media interest. The hospital or local authority should be able to initiate their own investigation. All of those involved should be aware that the police may also be contacted if allegation of a crime is made.

Those involved in such an event may suffer stress-related symptoms such as flashbacks, or difficulties in relating to family, friends or the environment. Feelings of fear and guilt are normal responses, even in those who were only peripherally involved. Staff should be made aware at the debriefing of the resources that are available to help them.

Other considerations

Many other recommendations, which are too numerous to list separately, exist to regulate the standards of various clinical environments. These govern aspects of the facilities such as the amount of space required, cleaning and infection control, the supply of utilities such as electricity and water, and the manufacturing standards of equipment. For example, an environment in which anaesthetic gases (e.g. nitrous oxide) are used must have an active gas-scavenging system in place, as Control of Substances Hazardous to Health (COSHH) recommendations govern the amount of contamination of the atmosphere by anaesthetic gases that is allowable.[23] These factors are not the direct responsibility of the sedationist, but the practitioner must be aware of their implications.

Other standards exist in relation to other equipment. For example, a dental chair must have the facility to be laid flat should an emergency occur, an operating table must be able to be tipped head down, suction apparatus must be available in case of potential aspiration, there must be a method of summoning emergency help, and so on.

The staffing of areas where sedation is given also requires careful consideration. When a general anaesthetic is being given, the minimum number of staff who should be present includes a surgeon, a scrub nurse, an anaesthetist, an anaesthetic assistant and a 'runner.' Guidance on the minimum number of staff who should be present for a sedation procedure is not so clear. A sedationist may also be the operator under some circumstances, but in such cases a separate person needs to be able to monitor the patient's condition, and intervene usefully if problems arise. There may also be a requirement to obtain extra equipment, help or facilities, so one could regard the minimum number of staff who should be present as at least three, namely the operator/ sedationist, the observer monitoring the patient, and a 'runner.' However, it is suggested that it is best practice in most circumstances if the sedationist and the operator are different people, and all staff members should be trained in appropriate life support measures.

Summary

It is safest to assume that the standards required for an environment where sedation is taking place should be similar to those for an operating theatre, as most of the recommendations have originated from anaesthetic professional bodies. It may be argued that when patients are being sedated for minor procedures or investigations, as opposed to being anaesthetised for operations, not all of these recommendations may be necessary. However, there is no evidence to show that sedation is inherently safer than anaesthesia per se, and so it should be assumed that a similar level of vigilance (irrespective of monitoring employed) should be exercised at all times in all circumstances. This chapter has identified some of the key considerations that a conscientious and professional sedationist must apply to their everyday practice.

LEARNING POINTS

- The safety of the patient is the paramount consideration.
- The sedationist must ensure that the environment is suitable for the procedure and sedation to occur.
- The sedationist should know what equipment is available, and be able to check it appropriately.
- Monitoring is a process, linking the patient's physiology to the observer.
- The observer must be able to interpret the parameters measured by the monitor appropriately, and formulate a proper action plan.
- Staff should be fully trained to deal with an emergency and its aftermath.

References

1 Blike G. Offsite anesthesiology: the challenge of seamless integration with non-anesthesiologist-delivered sedation/analgesia. *Curr Opin Anesthesiol.* 2007; **20:** 343–6.

2 Pino RM. The nature of anesthesia and procedural sedation outside of the operating room. *Curr Opin Anaesthesiol.* 2007; **20:** 347–51.

3 Royal College of Anaesthetists. *Anaesthesia in Remote Sites;* www.rcoa.ac.uk/docs/RemoteSites.pdf (accessed 13 April 2007).

4 Association of Anaesthetists of Great Britain and Ireland. *Checking Anaesthetic Equipment.* 3rd ed; www.aagbi.org/publications/guidelines/docs/checking04.pdf (accessed 15 April 2007).

5 Association of Anaesthetists of Great Britain and Ireland. *Standards for Monitoring During Anaesthesia and Recovery.* 4th ed; www.aagbi.org/publications/guidelines/docs/checking04.pdf (accessed 15 April 2007).

6 Weller J, Merry A, Warman G *et al.* Anaesthetists' management of oxygen pipeline failure: room for improvement. *Anaesthesia.* 2007; **62:** 122–6.

7 Semple P, Henrys P. Snippet: new species of cylinder. *Anaesthesia.* 2007; **62:** 428.

8 Wagstaff TAJ, Soni N. Performances of six types of oxygen delivery devices at varying respiratory rates. *Anaesthesia.* 2007; **62:** 492–503.

9 Cooper N. Acute care: treatment with oxygen; www.studentbmj.com/issues/04/02/education/56.php (accessed 15 April 2007).

10 Armstrong Davison MH. *The Evolution of Anaesthesia*. Altrincham: John Sherratt & Son; 1965.

11 Bryn Thomas K. *The Development of Anaesthetic Apparatus*. Oxford: Blackwell; 1975.

12 Keay S, Callander C. The safe use of infusion devices. *Contin Educ Anaesth Crit Care Pain*. 2004; **4:** 81–5.

13 National Patient Safety Agency. *Patient Safety Alert 21. Safer practice with epidural injections and infusions;* www.npsa.nhs.uk/display?contentId=5760 (accessed 4 August 2007).

14 Watkinson PJ, Barber VS, Price JD *et al.* A randomised controlled trial of the effect of continuous physiological monitoring on the adverse event rate in high-risk medical and surgical patients. *Anaesthesia*. 2006; **61:** 1031–40.

15 Association of Anaesthetists of Great Britain and Ireland. *Immediate Post-Anaesthetic Recovery;* www.aagbi.org/publications/guidelines/docs/checking04.pdf (accessed 15 April 2007).

16 Lightdale JR, Goldmann DA, Feldman HA *et al.* Microstream capnography improves patient monitoring during moderate sedation: a randomised controlled trial. *Pediatrics*. 2006; **117:** e1170–8.

17 Langton JA. Electrical safety. *R Coll Anaesth Newsletter*. 2000; **January issue:** 291.

18 Association of Anaesthetists of Great Britain and Ireland. *Anaphylactic Reactions Associated with Anaesthesia.* Revised ed; www.aagbi.org/publications/guidelines/docs/anaphylaxis03.pdf (accessed 23 May 2007).

19 www.lipidrescue.com

20 National Patient Safety Agency; www.npsa.nhs.uk/patientsafety/alerts-and-directives/alerts/epidural-injections-and-infusions/ (accessed 15 August 2007).

21 Association of Anaesthetists of Great Britain and Ireland. *Guidelines for the Management of Severe Local Anaesthetic Toxicity;* www.aagbi.org/publications/guidelines/docs/latoxicity07.pdf (accessed 3 September 2007).

22 Association of Anaesthetists of Great Britain and Ireland. *Catastrophes in Anaesthetic Practice: Dealing with the Aftermath;* www.aagbi.org/publications/guidelines/docs/catastrophes05.pdf (accessed 23 April 2007).

23 Health Services Advisory Committee. *Anaesthetic Agents: controlling exposure under COSSH.* London: Health Services Advisory Committee; 1995.

Further reading

Davey A, Moyle JTB, Ward CS. *Ward's Anaesthetic Equipment*. 5th ed. Oxford: WB Saunders; 2003.

Davis PD, Kenny GNC. *Basic Physics and Measurement in Anaesthesia*. 5th ed. Oxford: Butterworth-Heinemann; 2003.

CHAPTER 5

Drugs in sedation practice

A thorough understanding of the drugs that can be used for sedation, including their usual dosage, their safety profile, and their common interactions and side-effects, is essential to ensure patient safety. The sedationist must also understand the difference between drugs that are primarily used as sedatives, and those that are usually given for other purposes but which also have sedative side-effects. The aim of this chapter is to provide an introduction to the pharmacology of sedative medications, as well as describing some basic but important pharmacological principles.

Basic principles of pharmacology

Terms commonly used within this chapter are listed in Table 5.1.

TABLE 5.1 Definition of terms commonly used within this chapter

TERM	DEFINITION
Active site	The mechanism via which the drug will manifest its effect. The active site is usually, but not exclusively, part of a specific receptor.
Drug	A pharmacologically active substance.
Half-life	The time it takes for the concentration of the drug in the blood to decrease by 50%.
Main effect	A physiological or pharmacological action resulting from the administration of a drug, which is the intended effect.

cont.

TERM	DEFINITION
Receptor	A specific protein in a cell membrane to which the drug binds. Chemical changes within the cell are initiated which alter the activity of the cell, thereby exerting the drug's effect.
Side-effect	A physiological or pharmacological action resulting from the administration of a drug, which is not the intended main effect.
Therapeutic concentration	The concentration of a drug at which the therapeutic effects are manifested.
Therapeutic window	The difference between the therapeutic and toxic concentrations of a drug.
Toxic concentration	The concentration of a drug at which the risks from the side-effects outweigh the beneficial therapeutic effects of the drug.

Pharmacodynamics

This is the term used to describe the effects of the drug on the physiological processes of the body. A drug will only have an effect on a patient when it reaches its *active site*. The active site is usually, but not always, a specific protein receptor in a cell membrane. The drug interacts with the receptor, which then facilitates a change in the way that the cell functions. A cumulative effect from the altered activity in many cells will be manifested as a change in physiological system or organ activity.

Pharmacokinetics

Pharmacokinetics is the term used to describe the processes that determine the concentrations of a drug and its metabolites within the body.

In simple terms, in order to have the desired effect, the drug must be absorbed into or administered to the patient, transported to the receptor, and then perform an action at the active site. In order to end its effect, the drug must be removed from the active site, and then be removed from the body. Drugs are absorbed if they are administered directly to any part of the body other than the bloodstream. Thus medications given topically to skin and mucous membranes, or to the gastrointestinal system or intramuscularly, must usually (unless they are designed only to have an effect locally, such as a local anaesthetic) traverse membranes and enter the bloodstream.

In normal circumstances, the effect of the drug will increase as the amount of drug present at the active site increases. Unfortunately, it is not practicable to measure the concentration of a drug at the receptor, so the activity of a drug is usually related to its concentration in the blood. Drug dosages are calculated on the assumption that as a result of giving y mg to the patient, a concentration of x mg/ml will be present in the blood, and this will result in a set amount of drug being available at the active site, resulting in a predictable therapeutic effect.

The blood level at which the therapeutic effects are seen is called the *therapeutic concentration,* and the blood concentration at which undesirable effects are seen is called the *toxic concentration.* The difference between the two blood concentrations is called the *therapeutic window.* For an ideal drug, the therapeutic window would be very large – that is, the toxic concentration would be very much higher than the therapeutic concentration (*see* Figure 5.1). The larger the therapeutic window, the safer the drug is expected to be.

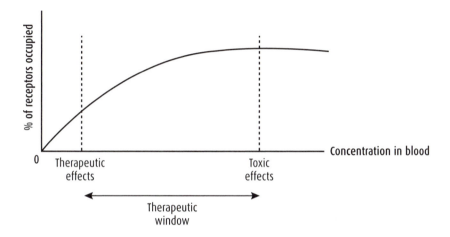

The concentration at which the drug therapeutic effects manifest is called the 'therapeutic concentration'. The concentration at which the toxic effects manifest is called the 'toxic concentration'. The 'therapeutic window' is the difference between these two concentrations, and will determine the 'safe' dosage of the drug.

FIGURE 5.1 The 'therapeutic window.'

Methods of drug administration

Drugs can be administered to the human body in a variety of different ways, each of which has advantages and disadvantages. These are summarised in Table 5.2.

The method of drug administration that is utilised will depend upon many factors related to the drug itself and the patient. For example, the formulation of the medication may determine that it is given intravenously rather than intramuscularly, or the patient may refuse to have the drug administered in a particular manner (e.g. they may decline a suppository but accept an injection).

TABLE 5.2 Different methods of drug administration

METHOD OF ADMINISTRATION		EXAMPLES	COMMENTS
Respiratory	Inhalational	Medical gases and vapours (e.g. anaesthetics, nitrous oxide, oxygen, etc.) can be administered in this manner. The drug enters the lungs, passes into the bloodstream, and is carried to the active site. The onset of effect will often require a set concentration of gas to be present in the lungs. This concentration will vary depending upon the gas or vapour used.	The main advantage is a rapid onset of effect, which is often but not exclusively coupled to a rapid offset. The amount used can easily be titrated to effect. Appropriate anaesthetic gas equipment is required. The facility to remove exhaled waste gases safely should be available.
Absorption across mucous membranes	Sublingual	The drug (e.g. sublingual glyceryl trinitrate for angina) passes through the mucous membrane of the mouth into the bloodstream, which carries it to the active site.	It is not possible to titrate the dose against the effect achieved.
	Nasal administration	The drug passes through the mucous membrane of the nose into the bloodstream, which carries it to the active site.	
	Oral	The drug is carried into the gastrointestinal system, where it can be absorbed into the bloodstream from a variety of sites.	Time to onset of effects will vary according to how long it takes the drug to reach the site of absorption in the gut. The drug is then subject to metabolism in the liver before it is carried to the active site. The effects can be unpredictable and are difficult to titrate.
	Rectal	The drug passes through the mucous membrane of the rectum into the bloodstream.	The use of rectal medication may not be acceptable to the patient. Specific consent is required.

cont.

METHOD OF ADMINISTRATION		EXAMPLES	COMMENTS
	Topical	The drug is absorbed through the skin.	The drug is initially absorbed into the subcutaneous tissue, where it forms a depot. It is then absorbed from the depot into the bloodstream. However, drugs can be designed to have a purely local effect (e.g. local anaesthetic medication).
Injection	Intramuscular	The drug is injected into the muscle.	It is necessary to avoid damaging important neighbouring tissues, such as nerves. Absorption can be unpredictable, due to alterations in blood flow.
	Intravenous	The drug is injected directly into the bloodstream.	Drug concentrations in the blood reach a high level very quickly. Drug dose can be titrated against effect.
	Subcutaneous	The drug is injected into the skin.	The drug is absorbed into the subcutaneous tissue, where it forms a depot. Unless it is designed to have a local effect (e.g. local anaesthetic), it is then absorbed from the depot into the bloodstream, and from there to the active site.

Ideally, a sedative drug will have a method of administration that is easy to use, and which will allow the effects of the drug to be manifested in a predictable and controllable manner. For this reason, in the majority of circumstances, sedation is given either by inhalation or by intravenous injection.

When a drug is being absorbed across a membrane, the rate of absorption is determined by the drug concentration at the site of administration. The greater the amount of drug, the faster the rate of absorption, and the higher the drug concentration in the blood will be.

In reality the situation is more complex, as the rate of absorption also depends upon factors such as drug solubility, molecular size and characteristics, tissue blood flow and any drug metabolism which occurs locally. Many drugs that are administered to the gastrointestinal system are subject to metabolism in the liver ('first pass' metabolism), thus reducing the concentration available systemically. Administering a drug directly to the bloodstream as an intravenous injection bypasses these factors, and so the resulting drug concentration in the blood may be higher than if the drug was given orally, but will also be achieved more rapidly.

This is illustrated in Figure 5.2. Clearly it may be very much more likely for a drug to reach the toxic concentration if it is given intravenously than if it is given by any other route. However, it is also easier to titrate the dose of the intravenous drug against the desired effect, because the effects produced by administering a small amount will be manifested quickly.

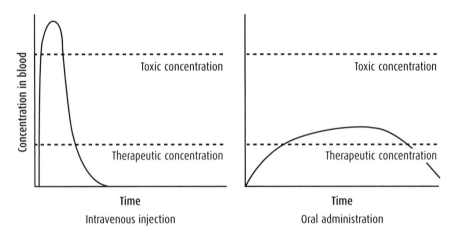

FIGURE 5.2 Drug concentration in the blood in relation to method of administration.

For the same reasons, the concentration of the drug in the bloodstream that is achieved by administering the drug orally may not be as consistent and predictable as when it is given intravenously. For example, if blood flow to the gastrointestinal mucosa is compromised, the rate of accumulation of an orally administered drug in the blood may be reduced, and it may therefore take longer to reach the therapeutic concentration. Alternatively, if the liver is functioning less efficiently, the rate of increase of the drug concentration in the blood may be faster than usual, and so may reach a higher level more quickly.

The concentration of a drug in the blood varies when repeated doses are given, depending upon the rate of removal and the frequency of administration of the drug. An intravenous bolus dose will result in the rapid attainment of a high concentration in the bloodstream, but administration of repeated doses of a drug at a rate faster than it is removed can result in accumulation, and eventual attainment of an equally high blood concentration, but after a more prolonged period. On the other hand, if the drug is given at infrequent intervals, the blood concentration may fall well below the therapeutic range before the next dose is given. This is illustrated in Figure 5.3.

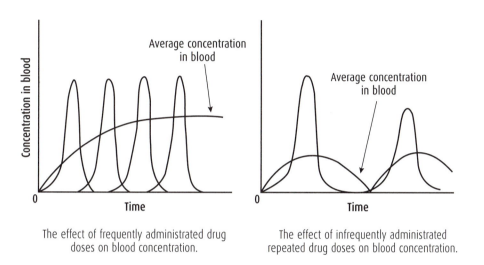

The effect of frequently administrated drug doses on blood concentration.

The effect of infrequently administrated repeated drug doses on blood concentration.

FIGURE 5.3 The effect of frequency of drug administration on average drug concentration in the blood.

However, if the drug can be given at the same rate as it is removed, the blood concentration will eventually reach an equilibrium, at which the level remains fairly constant. This situation occurs when a drug is given as an infusion.

Drug removal

Drugs can be removed from the body by a variety of mechanisms. Medical gases and vapours may simply be exhaled, some medications will be metabolised in body tissues before being excreted from the body, and other drugs may be excreted unchanged. The commonest site of drug metabolism is the liver, although other tissues may also be involved. The commonest routes of excretion are via the kidneys in the urine, or via the faeces.

The rate at which a drug is removed from the body usually remains constant under normal circumstances. In other words, over a set unit of time, the same proportion of drug will be removed. This rate of removal can be described in terms of the drug's *half-life* – that is, the time it takes for the concentration of the drug to be reduced by half. This is illustrated in Figure 5.4. A long half-life means that the drug is removed from the body very slowly, whereas a short half-life means that it is removed very quickly. It is important to remember that the half-life of a drug may vary from one patient to another. For instance, if a drug is metabolised in the liver, its half-life will be prolonged in a patient with liver impairment, or if it is eliminated via the kidneys, its half-life will be prolonged in a patient with kidney failure.

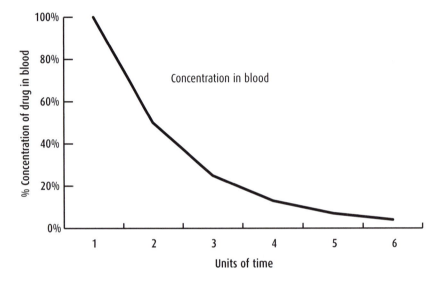

FIGURE 5.4 Half-life of a drug.

However, the duration of the therapeutic effects or side-effects of a drug may not be determined solely by the half-life. A drug will only exert an effect while it is at its active site. If the rate at which it is removed from the active site is dependent solely upon its metabolism, then the persistence of its effect will be dependent on the half-life of the drug – the longer the half-life, the longer the duration of action of the drug. However, if the drug is metabolised elsewhere, the persistence of its effects will be determined by other factors, such as how quickly it is removed from the active site. The anaesthetic drug propofol is a good example of this. It is short acting, because it is *redistributed* from the active site in the brain very quickly (within 1.3–4 minutes), whereas its *elimination* half-life is about 69 minutes. Therefore the desired effects of propofol wear off long before it is removed from the body. Other drugs may have permanent effects which do not wear off until tissues, receptors or physiological processes are regenerated. Drug effects that persist long after they are useful are sometimes referred to as *'hangover effects.'* Box 5.1 summarises the pharmacological principles discussed so far.

BOX 5.1 Summary of pharmacological principles

- Drugs can be administered in a variety of ways, but usually need to reach a specific active site in order to exert their effects.
- Blood concentration is used as a measure of drug concentration at the active site.
- Various factors affect the rate at which the total concentration is achieved, and the final concentration reached. These will be dependent upon the method of drug administration.
- Intravenous drug administration can result in higher blood concentrations of the drug being attained more quickly, but it is relatively easy to titrate the dose of the drug against the desired effect.
- The rate at which a drug's effects wear off are not always the same as the rate at which the drug is removed from the body.

The pharmacology of sedatives

It is essential that the sedationist remembers that all sedatives are in fact *central nervous system depressants*. This means that they will depress consciousness and body protective reflexes, as well as respiratory and cardiovascular function. As such the therapeutic window may be very narrow, and may be reduced much further by concomitant drug therapy.

In order to better understand the effects of different sedative agents, it is best to first determine what characteristics the 'ideal sedative' should possess. By comparing available drugs with the ideal, it is easy to determine the advantages and drawbacks of a particular drug in a particular situation.

Characteristics of the ideal sedative agent

Some characteristics of the ideal sedative drug are listed in Table 5.3.

The ideal sedative would be safe to use, predictable in its effects, short acting, and would not persist in the body, but would produce inactive metabolites that are easily excreted. It would have a large therapeutic window, and its effects could be reversed by a specific antidote in the event of accident.

Drugs that are used specifically to provide sedation can be categorised into two broad groups, namely benzodiazepines and anaesthetic agents.

TABLE 5.3 Characteristics of the ideal sedative drug

Versatility	Ability to be administered to the patient by a variety of different routes.
	Acceptability to patients.
Actions	Predictable and reproducible therapeutic effect.
	Rapid onset and offset of effect.
	No 'hangover' effect.
	Wide safety margin.
	Existence of a specific antidote.
	Useful additional effects (e.g. analgesia, amnesia, etc.).
Other characteristics	Cheap.
	Easily storable, with long shelf-life.
	Pharmacologically and physiologically inactive metabolites.

Benzodiazepines

Benzodiazepines are a ubiquitous family of drugs whose effects include hypnosis, sedation, anxiolysis, amnesia, relief of muscular tension and anticonvulsive properties. They are thought to act via specific receptors at nerve synapses in the central nervous system that are particularly plentiful in the cortex and midbrain. These receptors are believed to be mediated by gamma-amino butyric acid (GABA). It is thought that they facilitate the influx of chloride ions into neurons, hyperpolarising the cells and preventing the transmission of electrical nerve impulses in response to normal stimuli. This results in the depression of the central nervous system.

Benzodiazepines are also associated with depression of cardiorespiratory parameters, reflexes and responses. The broad range of depressive effects accounts for most of the listed adverse reactions, apart from those specific to a particular formulation or mode of administration. A specific antidote to benzodiazepines exists, namely *flumazenil (Anexate)*. Paradoxical excitement can occur with the use of benzodiazepines.

Midazolam is a commonly available water-soluble intravenous benzodiazepine. The end point that indicates successful sedation is drowsiness and slurring of speech. It is popular not only because of the ease of administration, but also because of the reputed amnesic effects. Although formulated for intravenous use, it can be given orally or nasally if correctly prepared.

However, it should be used with caution, particularly in the elderly, as the dose required to produce anaesthesia is not that different to the dose required for sedation. Midazolam has been used in anaesthetic practice to induce anaesthesia at doses of 0.8 mg/kg as a bolus. An 80-kg man would therefore require only 6.5 mg as a bolus to induce anaesthesia. It is recommended that the drug is given in small doses, titrated to effect. Midazolam has been subject to specific cautions recommended by the National Confidential Enquiry into Patient Outcome and Death (NCEPOD).[1]

Diazepam is not water soluble, and so is commonly presented in a lipid emulsion as *Diazemuls* for use in sedation for procedures. Oral and rectal formulations also exist and are absorbed rapidly. The quoted intravenous dose is 10–20 mg, but it is prudent to administer it incrementally until the desired effect is achieved. Diazepam is metabolised in the liver to active metabolites (including temazepam) which have long half-lives (in some cases over 100 hours).

Temazepam is commonly used as a treatment for anxiety and insomnia, and as a premedication by anaesthetists. It is available in syrup and tablet form.

Lorazepam is available in oral and intravenous/intramuscular formulations. It has a longer duration of action than diazepam. It is often used as an anticonvulsant in emergencies.

Flumazenil is a specific antidote to the effects of benzodiazepines, competing with the latter to bind to the active site (competitive antagonism). The drug is formulated as 100 µg per ml solution. It is recommended that in the case of suspected benzodiazepine overdose this drug is given incrementally, 100 µg at a time, until the patient shows signs of recovery. The maximum dose for an adult in most circumstances is 1 mg, but the user must be aware that administration to a known epileptic may produce convulsions by reversing the beneficial anticonvulsive effect of benzodiazepines. In some circumstances flumazenil may be given as an infusion.

As the use of flumazenil suggests that an overdose of benzodiazepine has been given, the patient should be subject to careful post-administrative observation. Because the effects of flumazenil may not persist as long as those of the benzodiazepine whose effects it is reversing, re-sedation is a real possibility. Side-effects include flushing, nausea, vomiting, hypertension, anxiety and headache. Flumazenil is metabolised in the liver to inert compounds which are excreted in the urine.

Anaesthetic agents

Inhalational anaesthetic agents

Inhalational anaesthetic agents are subdivided into two groups, namely the anaesthetic gas nitrous oxide, and the anaesthetic vapours.

Nitrous oxide (N_2O) is commonly presented either as the pure gas (in blue pressurised cylinders) or as *Entonox*, a 50/50 mixture with oxygen (in blue cylinders with a white and black shoulder). Some work has been performed, mainly in obstetric practice, with other formulations in which Entonox is mixed with an anaesthetic vapour, such as isoflurane (*Isonox*).

Nitrous oxide is stored as a pressurised gas over a liquid form. As such, the gauge pressure of the cylinder will not start to fall below 'full' until the liquid phase has been used up completely. This means that when the gauge pressure does start to fall, the cylinder is virtually empty and will soon need to be replaced. The gas is not inflammable but will support combustion. Common side-effects include nausea and vomiting.

Nitrous oxide has a pleasant smell, and is well tolerated by patients of all ages. Its main effect is analgesic, possibly mediated via opiate receptors, but it also provides some sedation, as it is a central nervous system depressant. It has a rapid onset, and the effects wear off within several normal breaths after the supply is removed. The gas is not very soluble in blood, and rapidly moves into air-filled spaces such as the middle ear, the bowel, emphysematous bullae and pneumothoraces, which can be hazardous. Its use is contraindicated after retinal surgery in which a gas bubble has been used to secure retinal re-attachment, as nitrous oxide influx into the bubble can cause an increase in intra-ocular pressure, and blindness.

Nitrous oxide is not metabolised, but prolonged exposure can have toxic effects. These include anaemia and peripheral neuropathy. In addition, nitrous oxide may be teratogenic in early pregnancy. The maximum allowable atmospheric level over an 8-hour period is 100 parts per million under COSHH regulations.[2]

Nitrous oxide should not be used for sedation in less than 30% oxygen. If it is being administered via an anaesthetic machine (Boyle's machine), it is incumbent on the sedationist to ensure that a hypoxic mixture is not being administered.

Anaesthetic vapours such as *halothane, enflurane, isoflurane* and *sevoflurane* are volatile hydrocarbon liquids that rapidly vaporise at room temperatures. *Desflurane* is a similar agent which needs to be given via a special heated vaporiser. These vapours should only be administered by anaesthetically trained staff. They all have a pungent smell and are very powerful global central nervous system depressants, although the mechanism of action has not been fully elucidated. These agents are subject to varying degrees of metabolism in the liver. Halothane in particular has been associated with development of an inflammatory hepatitis in susceptible individuals. All of the vapours are possible triggers for malignant hyperthermia, a genetic condition in which sensitive individuals become hypermetabolic on exposure to certain medications, resulting in high temperature, muscle dysfunction and acidosis. If left untreated, the condition is fatal, but it is rapidly reversible using *dantrolene*. Sevoflurane and desflurane are commonly utilised for day-case anaesthesia. They are all subject to COSSH regulation.

Dantrolene is a muscle relaxant which works by interfering with calcium metabolism in muscles. When it is used to treat malignant hyperthermia, large amounts may be required. It can cause sedation and muscle weakness, and should only be utilised by those skilled in its administration.

Intravenous anaesthetic agents
Barbiturates

Barbiturates are central nervous system depressants which are thought to act both by reducing neurotransmitter release and by reducing neurotransmitter-receptor sensitivity. They are commonly used to induce anaesthesia and in the treatment of status epilepticus. They are not usually used for sedation, as the therapeutic window is quite small. Their use must be avoided in patients known to have porphyria.

Thiopentone is the most commonly available barbiturate in anaesthetic practice. It must be reconstituted from powder for intravenous use, and is stored in ampoules under nitrogen gas. It causes profound respiratory and cardiovascular depression. Extravasation can cause pain and sometimes tissue necrosis, as the solution is very alkaline. Accidental arterial injection can be disastrous, causing limb ischaemia. It is occasionally used in the short term as an infusion in ITU situations.

Methohexitone is also reconstituted from powder, and again is a very alkaline solution.

Non-barbiturates

Propofol is a phenol derivative which is suspended in a lipid emulsion. The lipid emulsion contains soy and egg protein. It can be used intravenously as a bolus, an infusion or via a patient-controlled sedation (PCS) device. It is not clear exactly how it exerts its effects. Injection can be associated with pain, which can be alleviated by including small amounts of local anaesthetic in the mixture. It is a central nervous system depressant, and as such depresses respiration, the cardiovascular system and protective airway reflexes. It is commonly used to sedate ITU patients, and is the agent of choice for total intravenous anaesthesia (TIVA). It has a rapid onset and offset, and may be associated with vivid, pleasant (and sometimes sexual) dreams. It is metabolised in the liver. The anaesthetic dose is 1.5–2.5 mg/kg as a bolus. Smaller doses can be used to provide sedation.

In TIVA, the drug can be administered as an infusion using a specialist syringe driver. Originally, the operator placed a set concentration of propofol (e.g. 1% or 2%) in a 50-ml syringe, and set a rate of ml/hour or ml/ minute. The operator had to constantly monitor the patient and the pump, and titrate the administration rate against the patient's level of anaesthesia. This technique has been refined in recent years to one of target-controlled infusion (TCI), the 'target' being the concentration of propofol in the blood or at the active site. The operator programmes the pump with the patient's age, weight and other relevant data, and sets a blood concentration level to be achieved. Using the patient parameters that have been programmed in, the pump calculates the rate required to reach this blood level. A plasma concentration of 0.5–1.5 µg/ml is associated with sedation, and a level above 4 µg/ml is associated with anaesthesia. A variety of patient controlled sedation (PCS) techniques have been described.[3] In PCS, the infusion pump delivers a set amount of propofol for a set time when the patient presses a demand button. The device is programmed with both a dose limit (so that only a maximum dose of propofol can be delivered over a set time) and a time lock-out function (e.g. so that only one dose can be given every 3 minutes). In the UK, it is not recommended that these methods are used by non-anaesthetists. It is important that the pumps are not allowed to be used for other purposes, as unskilled personnel may not understand that the delivery rate can be programmed in a variety of ways (*see* Box 5.2).

BOX 5.2 Importance of understanding the infusion pump

Anaesthetic staff were called to a ward during the night because a patient had become extremely drowsy. The patient had undergone a routine operation 2 days previously, but had been complaining of pain. The ward staff had commenced a morphine infusion, but had used a TIVA pump from theatre in error. Instead of a rate of 'ml/hour', the pump had been set to deliver 'ml/minute', as staff had been unaware that the units used could be changed. The patient made a full recovery.

Etomidate is an imidazole, presented as a liquid, which is used to induce anaesthesia. Its use as infusions on ITU was stopped after it was associated with an excess number of deaths due to steroid depression.

Ketamine is a phencyclidine derivative, presented in a liquid form in a variety of concentrations. It can be used intravenously or intramuscularly, and appears to work through an N-methyl d-aspartate (NMDA)-mediated receptor. Unlike the other anaesthetic agents, it causes sympathetic nervous system stimulation, resulting in increased blood pressure and heart rate. It also has analgesic properties. It increases respiratory rate, but may still depress airway protective reflexes. Its main advantage over other agents is its profound analgesic effect. However, it is associated with increased nausea and vomiting, and very vivid, unpleasant hallucinations. It is recommended that a benzodiazepine is also administered to reduce the effects of the latter. It also increases salivation, which is potentially dangerous as it can be associated with choking and bronchospasm. Ketamine is broken down in the liver to active metabolites.

Safety profile

The possible complications associated with these different drugs vary in type and frequency. A recent review of sedation in American emergency departments suggested that the incidence of respiratory depression with propofol was 50%, compared with an incidence of 33% with etomidate, for example, although it was recognised that the use of propofol resulted in superior procedural conditions.[4] The local department in which sedation is being performed should develop a guideline that determines what sedation can be administered, and by what means. However, the sedationist should use their knowledge of pharmacology to determine the best single sedative or combination, in order to ensure patient safety and procedural success.

Other drugs that are used as sedatives

Many other drugs of different types are also used as sedatives. Chloral hydrate, triclofos, antihistamines and melatonin are all used as oral sedatives in paediatric practice, and are covered in more detail in Chapter 7.

Drugs with sedative side-effects

Many drugs cause sedation as an unintended side-effect. The effect can be unpredictable, so these medications should not be given with the primary intention of providing sedation. If given simultaneously with sedative drugs, there is a possibility of accidentally achieving a deeper level of sedation than intended, with resulting hazards to the patient. Many of the procedures for which sedation is necessary are painful, and require a degree of pain relief. Sedatives are therefore commonly given in combination with analgesic medication, and many analgesics are known to have sedative effects.

Opiate analgesics

These commonly utilised analgesics are thought to exert their effects through specific receptors spread throughout the body. The main opiate receptor is termed the mu-receptor. It is thought that opiate receptors allow cells to become hyperpolarised, reducing the excitability of cell membranes. This prevents the transmission of electrical nerve impulses triggered by painful stimuli. Opiates have many supplementary effects, due to the ubiquitous distribution of the mu-receptors. Cardiovascular effects include bradycardia and hypotension. Opiates are known to be potent depressants of respiration and protective airway reflexes. They are also associated with nausea, vomiting, itchiness and constipation.

Morphine is available in a variety of preparations and can be administered orally, nasally (if correctly formulated), intramuscularly or intravenously. It is metabolised in the liver, and excreted mainly in the urine.

Diamorphine is metabolised in the liver, producing morphine as a metabolite. It is therefore more potent than morphine. It exists in a variety of forms and can be administered either by injection or orally.

Pethidine is not as potent as morphine. It can be administered orally, intravenously or intramuscularly, and may accumulate in renal impairment. It is subject to specific cautions relating to its use in the elderly.[1]

Fentanyl, alfentanil, sufentanil and remifentanil are exceedingly potent intravenous opiates. They are best regarded as anaesthetic drugs, and their use by non-anaesthetists is not recommended. They are generally short acting, but are very powerful respiratory depressants. Remifentanil has a very short duration of action, and is commonly given as an infusion rather than as a bolus.

Naloxone is a specific opiate antagonist that is used to reverse the effects of opiate medication. It competes with opiates to bind inactively at the mu-receptors. It is usually presented as a 400 µg/ml phial, and should be given in small increments titrated to effect in order to counter respiratory depression. It can be given intravenously or intramuscularly, and it can also be given as an infusion. The necessity for using naloxone suggests that an overdose of opiates has occurred, and as its duration of action is commonly shorter than that of the drug it is counteracting, the patient will require careful observation to ensure that unnoticed re-sedation does not occur. The user should also be aware that if naloxone is used in opiate-dependent patients it may induce an acute withdrawal syndrome. It has no common major side-effects, but has rarely been reported to be associated with cardiac arrhythmia. It is extensively metabolised in the liver.

Other relevant drugs

The sedationist will need to be familiar with many drugs which, although they may have no immediate relevance to the act of sedation, may be utilised by other staff during the procedure that the patient is undergoing, and which have potential for causing either side-effects or drug interactions which the sedationist will be expected to treat.

Local anaesthetic agents

Local anaesthetic agents work by blocking sodium channels in nervous tissue, thereby preventing the propagation of nerve impulses. They can be administered either topically or by injection. They are used to provide analgesia to a relatively localised area (e.g. a particular patch of skin, the oropharynx, etc.) or to a particular nerve supply (e.g. blocking a particular nerve or group of nerves), or to provide surgical anaesthesia (e.g. as an intrathecal or epidural injection). The local anaesthetic solution may contain a variety of substances, including adrenaline, preservatives and antimicrobial agents. Local anaesthetic agents can be cardiotoxic, leading to cardiac arrhythmias that are resistant to treatment. This can result from overdosage, or it can be caused by accidental administration of a local anaesthetic into the bloodstream.

Local anaesthetic toxicity is indicated by oral tingling, agitation, cardio-vascular collapse, respiratory arrest and fitting, and may be fatal. It has been suggested that administration of a lipid solution intravenously could have an antidote effect in these circumstances. Local anaesthetics include lidocaine (lignocaine), bupivacaine, cinchocaine, cocaine and prilocaine.

Antihistamines

Antihistamine-type drugs have a variety of actions, one of which is sedation. These medications are commonly used in the sedation of children, as they can be given orally.

Anaesthetic muscle relaxants

Muscle relaxants are not sedatives, and should only be used as part of an anaesthetic technique by an anaesthetist. They interfere with the transmission of nerve impulses to and through muscle tissue, resulting in total paralysis. Without artificial ventilation the patient would die from hypoxia. Muscle relaxants include atracurium, vecuronium, suxamethonium and rocuronium.

Summary

Sedative drugs have a wide variety of chemical structures, but have the common effect of being central nervous system depressants. Their use by the unskilled can therefore be particularly hazardous. Sedationists should regularly check their own hospital formulary, or national sources, to ensure that drug licensing or dosage recommendations have not changed.

LEARNING POINTS

- Drugs with *sedative effects* are not the same as *sedative drugs*.
- Sedationists need to understand pharmacological principles, as these will guide their decision making with regard to choice of technique and choice of drug used.
- No one single sedative drug will be ideal for every situation.
- Although some drugs have specific antidotes, many do not. The use of a specific antidote implies that overdosage has occurred, and the patient will require specific observation.

References

1 Gray A, Bell GD. Elderly patients vulnerable because of excessive doses of sedatives; www.ncepod.org.uk/pdf/current/NPSA%20sedation%20article.pdf (accessed 2 February 2007).

2 Health Services Advisory Committee. *Anaesthetic Agents: controlling exposure under COSHH.* London: Health Services Advisory Committee; 1995.

3 Barakat AR, Sutcliffe N, Schwab M. Effect site concentration during propofol TCI sedation: a comparison of sedation scores with two pharmacokinetic models. *Anaesthesia.* 2007; **62:** 661–7.

4 Smalley AJ, Nowicki TA. Sedation in the Emergency Department. *Curr Opin Anaesthesiol.* 2007; **20:** 379–83.

Further reading

electronic Medicines Compendium (eMC); http://emc.medicines.org.uk

Royal Pharmaceutical Society of Great Britain. *British National Formulary No. 52 (September 2006).* London: BMJ Publishing Group; 2006 (updated every 6 months).

Hladky SB. *Pharmacokinetics.* Manchester: Manchester University Press; 1990.

Sasada M, Smith S. *Drugs in Anaesthesia and Intensive Care.* 3rd ed. Oxford: Oxford Medical Publications; 2003.

CHAPTER 6

Medico-legal aspects of sedation

Healthcare workers must have a good understanding of the basic legal framework within which they practise, including knowledge of the regulatory, statutory and ethical standards which govern their activities. This chapter will *not* provide an exhaustive analysis of the potential legal pitfalls relating to sedation, but it will give a brief outline of the common concepts of which sedationists should be aware.

Consent

Consent to treatment is a vital tool in medical practice. The *Oxford Popular English Dictionary* defines 'consent' as to *'agree, give permission.'*[1] However, in medico-legal terms, the word suggests a much more complex paradigm, describing a process of understanding between patient and healthcare provider rather than a mere passive agreement to treatment. Medical consent is now often referred to as *informed consent*, and has evolved as a concept over many years.[2,3]

Modern thinking with regard to consent in the Western world was shaped in the aftermath of the Nuremberg trials of Nazi doctors involved in human medical experimentation.[4] These trials set an international standard for the consent of patients who participate in research, and subsequently influenced the consent process throughout the health sector.

In simple terms, the consent of the patient is required not only before any treatment can be given, but also before the practitioner can even touch the patient. In British law, any health practitioner who does not obtain consent before handling or treating the patient can be guilty of *assault* (an act which causes the person subjected to it an apprehension of the immediate infliction of a battery) or *battery* (the physical use of force on another's person).

Implied and explicit consent

The term '*implied consent*' describes the situation in which the patient gives consent by their actions. Examples of such situations include a phlebotomist asking to take some blood, and the patient holding their arm out and not protesting, or the dentist asking to examine the patient's teeth, and the patient sitting in the dental chair and opening their mouth. However, some procedures are complex, invasive or involve intimacy, and it should not be assumed that implied consent will apply in these cases. For example, although the patient with toothache may well expect the dentist to place instruments inside their mouth when they sit in the dental chair, it should not be assumed that they also consent to the insertion of a painkilling suppository after treatment[5] (*see* Box 6.1). In addition, some treatments may have possible consequences for the individual involved. In these cases, it is advisable to gain the *explicit consent* of the patient. Explicit consent is taken to mean that a discussion took place with the patient, detailing the procedure, the possible side-effects or complications that might result, and also the consequences of not undergoing the procedure, and what alternatives are available. In order for the consent to be fully informed, the patient must be able to consider properly the risks and benefits of the procedure before reaching their decision.

BOX 6.1 Failure to obtain proper consent

X, a 22-year-old woman, had four teeth extracted under general anaesthesia at a community dental surgery. The experienced anaesthetist, Dr Z, inserted an analgesic suppository while X was anaesthetised. Unfortunately, Dr Z inserted the suppository vaginally. The patient alleged that a sexual assault had taken place. This was proven not to be the case, but Dr Z was referred to the GMC for failing to obtain specific consent for suppository use. The dentist was referred to the GDC. The GMC accepted that the use of a painkilling suppository was good practice, but found Dr Z guilty of serious professional misconduct for not obtaining specific consent, and therefore guilty of an assault. He received an admonishment.

Mitchell JA. Fundamental problem of consent. *BMJ.* 1995; **310**: 43–6.
Laljee MMA. Dentist is aggrieved at outcome. *BMJ.* 1995; **310**: 935.

Contrary to popular belief, consent does not necessarily require obtaining the signature of a patient on a form, and in fact a signed consent form itself may mean very little under the law, other than at some point a person has signed a piece of paper. What is important from a legal point of view is that the practitioner has recorded the details of the discussion and the consent process.[6]

There are several prerequisites that must hold true for consent to be valid.

Capacity

The patient must have the *capacity* to give consent. An individual has a fundamental right of autonomy – that is, the right to determine what does, or does not, happen to them. The Mental Capacity Act (2005) has enshrined this principle in British law. The adult patient is always assumed to have the capacity to give or withhold their consent unless it can be proved otherwise. Simply making a decision which the medical or nursing practitioner believes to be unwise cannot be taken to mean that the patient lacks capacity. Capacity can be a difficult issue to address, as it can be decision specific – that is, there may be some decisions which it is felt the patient has the capacity to make, and others which it is felt that they do not.

In order to make an informed decision, the patient must be able to understand information which is given to them, and have the ability to consider it, to use it to make a decision, and then to be able to communicate that decision. However, lack of ability to communicate on its own may not necessarily indicate lack of capacity. It may be that practitioners believe that the patient permanently lacks capacity (e.g. due to dementia) or temporarily lacks capacity (e.g. due to delirium), in which case they are obliged to take treatment decisions on the basis of what they believe is in the *best interests* of the patient. Best interests can be determined by consulting the records, any existing advance directives, and the patient's relatives or partner. In some circumstances, the patient may have appointed a legally confirmed, designated decision maker, who has a *lasting power of attorney (LPA)*, to make decisions on their behalf if they become incompetent. The final decision as to whether to provide treatment or not will always be that of the healthcare team. However, the team must understand that their judgement and decisions might be challenged at a future date.

In summary, only a competent adult can give consent for him- or herself to undergo treatment. If they are incapable of giving consent, another adult *cannot* normally give consent for them, although the relatives and next of kin can be consulted to determine what the patient's wishes may have been. If there is disagreement between the family and the treating health practitioners as to what the patient's best interests may be, the healthcare staff may have to resort to the Courts for a determination. The ability of healthcare staff to determine 'best interests' for an adult who does not have capacity have recently been challenged in law (*see* Box 6.2).

> ### BOX 6.2 Challenge to the ability of medical staff to determine the patient's best interests
>
> In 2002, the GMC produced guidance for doctors with regard to end-of-life scenarios.[7] Mr B suffered from a progressive neurological disorder and believed that the document gave doctors the inviolable right to stop hydration and nutrition for him if he became unable to express his views, effectively allowing him to starve to death or die of thirst. Mr B subsequently challenged the guidance in Court under the Human Rights Act (1998), and won. However, the decision was overturned in the Court of Appeal. The case did successfully highlight how the autonomy of individuals should be respected, and how patients and the carers of those with debilitating and progressive diseases should ensure that all aspects of their treatment are discussed, including detailed end-of-life scenarios.
>
> *Burke v GMC* [2004] EWHC 1879.

The situation with regard to children is more complex. Briefly, consent is normally required from a parent or guardian, but a child can give consent if they are judged to be '*Gillick competent*' (*Gillick v West Norfolk and Wisbech Health Authority* [1985] 3 All ER 402). However, a child under the age of majority, even if they are Gillick competent, cannot normally refuse consent to treatment.

Consent must be voluntary

When giving consent, patients must not perceive themselves to be under any kind of duress that could adversely influence their capacity to make a reasoned decision. They must have been given adequate time to consider the options and to weigh up the information that they have received. For example, consent taken in the operating theatre seconds before a procedure is to start may not be regarded as valid on these grounds.

Appropriate information must have been provided

The standard of information required to be given to the patient, particularly with regard to risks, must be felt to be appropriate, although what detail is felt to be adequate is not subject to set rules. The standard utilised in law is that of what the *'prudent patient'* rather than the *'prudent doctor'* feels is necessary. This was a concept first enshrined in the USA (*Salgo v Leland* [1957]). For example, an anaesthetist may not normally mention to most patients the small chance of vocal cord damage and resultant voice changes occurring during endotracheal intubation. However, if the patient is a professional opera singer, this information might well be judged to be extremely important. In the Sidaway case (*Sidaway v Bethlehem Royal Hospital* [1985] AL 871 HL), a doctor was found not to have been negligent in failing to disclose a risk of spinal cord damage during a neck operation, because his practice was in accordance with a responsible body of neurosurgical opinion at the time. However, as the landmark case described in Box 6.3 shows, this may not hold true all the time.

BOX 6.3 Lack of information given for informed consent

Miss C had had back problems for a number of years, and was referred to a neurosurgeon, Mr A. She underwent spinal surgery, but suffered complications and was paralysed. She subsequently sued Mr A. The Court accepted that Mr A had not been negligent in performing the surgery. However, they ruled that despite this, Miss C should be awarded damages because the consent process had been flawed. They believed that Mr A had not appropriately emphasised the small risk of paralysis. Had he done so, Miss C might well have deferred surgery while she obtained more information, and the complication might not have occurred. This decision was upheld on appeal.

Chester v Afshar [2004] UKHL 41.
www.publications.parliament.uk/pa/ld200304/ldjudgmt/jd041014/cheste-2.htm (accessed 18 April 2007).

Anaesthesia is an area of practice in which, until recently, the concept of consent has been vague. In fact, anaesthesia was often regarded as a mere adjunct to surgery. Nowadays, however, it is advised that anaesthetists should discuss the risks and benefits of the anaesthetic with the patient, and record this discussion appropriately.[8-10] In this respect, sedation is no different from anaesthesia, as it has distinct and defined consequences for the patient which are separate to those of the proposed medical intervention that it facilitates. It therefore follows that separate consent for sedation should also be obtained.

Although it is best practice for the person who will be performing the procedure to obtain the patient's consent, this is not always necessary. Consent can be obtained some time beforehand by a trained individual (i.e. someone who is capable of discussing the procedure with the patient appropriately), but the patient's consent must be checked by those performing the procedure when the patient returns for the operation. In other words, the onus is on the sedationist to be secure in their own mind that the patient has given appropriate, informed consent.

This requires that the patient has been adequately informed about the sedative techniques which are to be employed, what the benefits and side-effects might be, and what the alternatives are (e.g. non-pharmacological options). The sedationist should always enquire as to whether there are any personal or religious reasons why the patient may not want sedation. For example, Scientologists may not wish to be sedated at all. In addition, it must be clear that the patient understands the consequences of not having the sedation, or of opting for the alternative technique. Finally, the sedationist must ensure that the patient is aware of the activities that they must not engage in following the sedation, such as operating machinery, being left alone, being left in charge of under-age children, driving, signing legal documentation, and so on. If the sedationist is also performing the operative procedure, it must be clear that the consent issues relating to sedation are different from those relating to the procedure itself.

Standards of practice

In modern healthcare practice, many tasks that were previously the sole remit of doctors and dentists are now being performed by a variety of professionals, including nursing staff, physiotherapists and new technician roles. In the UK, unlike many parts of Europe and the USA, there has never been a role for the *nurse anaesthetist*, although several pilot studies have recently been commissioned and have yet to report. However, there has long been established a role for the *nurse practitioner* performing medical procedures such as endoscopy, and providing the sedation for their own procedures or those of others.

The question then arises as to whether the standard of practice expected of these non-medical staff is the same as that expected of a doctor. If so, how experienced a doctor would that be? Or is it in fact a different standard of practice, and if it is different, is it lower?

To some extent this question has already been addressed in British case law (*see* Box 6.4).

> **BOX 6.4 Expected standards of practice**
>
> A premature baby had a catheter placed into the wrong blood vessel by a paediatric senior house officer (SHO), which meant that incorrect blood results were used to guide oxygen therapy, resulting in brain damage. The SHO had not recognised the misplacement, nor had the registrar who had been asked to check the catheter's position. The SHO was found not guilty of negligence because they had recognised the limits of their knowledge and referred to a more experienced doctor to check the line's position. The registrar was found guilty of negligence, for failing to recognise the problem, which is something that a practitioner of their professed level of skill should have identified.
>
> *Wilsher v Essex Health Authority* [1986] 3 All ER 801.

There are several standards that could be applied to practice in this regard.

The team standard of practice

This concept suggests that everyone in a particular healthcare team must work to the same standard. The difficulty is that this would assume that, for example, an experienced nurse, a newly qualified doctor and a professor of surgery who all work in the same team would be expected to have the same knowledge, experience and utility.

An individualised standard of practice

This suggests that the standard applied will depend only upon an individual's particular training and experience, and that it is not possible to define a uniform standard of care unless everyone has exactly the same skill and competency.

The standard of practice required of the environment/post

This is the standard preferred in British law. A person who works as, for example, a registrar in gastroenterology would be expected to work to the standard which was reasonable for someone who was competent in that role. In other words, the patient has a right to expect that someone perform-ing a particular skilled job is furnished with a minimum level of skill, and is able to apply a minimum, defined standard of care. However, this does not make any allowance for the post holder making an error because of inexperience. Even if it is your first day as a sedationist, you are expected to act with skill reasonable for a person trained in giving sedation. It is for the individual to recognise the limitations of their skill and experience, and to seek senior assistance or advice when they feel that they cannot act with reasonable care.

This does not mean that all sedationists should demonstrate exactly the same skills and utility as an anaesthetist, simply because some anaesthetists will perform sedation. However, it does mean that they will have to demonstrate that they are able to provide a minimum standard of care, and have appropriate skills, *some* of which will clearly overlap with those of an anaesthetist. These skills have been outlined very clearly in some subspecialties – for example, with regard to dental practice by the Dental Sedation Teachers Group (DSTG). It has been recommended that the skills and techniques that are safe for use in particular clinical circumstances should be defined by relevant Royal Colleges or associations.[11] However, the general skill sets for sedationists should be the same irrespective of the specialty in which they trained, their healthcare discipline, or the procedure for which they are providing sedation (*see* Chapter 2).

Negligence

In law, negligence has a specific meaning.
➡ There must have been a duty of care.
➡ That duty of care must have been breached.
➡ The breach in the duty of care must have been responsible for harm to the patient occurring as a result.

This is referred to as the chain of 'causation', and for a claim of negligence to be upheld, all links in the chain must be proved. In the UK, case law in relation to negligence is based upon the so-called Bolam test (*Bolam v Friern Hospital Management Committee* [1957] 1 WLR 582). In essence, the test suggests that the health professional must provide treatment to a standard which is recognised as proper by a responsible body of other health professionals. However, this does not imply that the treatment must necessarily be what the majority do. The Law was further refined by the Bolitho ruling (*Bolitho v City and Hackney Health Authority* [1997] 3 WLR

1151). It is possible for the Court to prefer the opinion of one responsible body of professionals over another, in essence deciding whether actions suggested as acceptable by a body of medical opinion were in fact reasonable under the individual circumstances presented.

These cases are summarised in Box 6.5.

BOX 6.5 Practice in accordance with a responsible body of professional opinion

A patient underwent electroconvulsive therapy treatment, but was not given muscle relaxant, and suffered serious injury during the resultant convulsions. It was argued that it was negligent not to have administered muscle relaxant. However, it was accepted that a responsible body of medical opinion believed that not giving the relaxant was reasonable practice, due to the complications and side-effects that could result from the drug.

Bolam v Friern Hospital Management Committee [1957] 1 WLR 582.

A child had a cardiac arrest and developed brain damage in hospital. He had suffered previous episodes of breathing difficulty but, despite being informed about them, the paediatric registrar did not review the patient. Although a breach of duty was found, it was not clear whether causation was provable, as expert evidence argued that several different courses of action were open to the registrar, all of which were reasonable, some of which would have made no difference to the outcome.

Bolitho v City and Hackney Health Authority [1997] 3 WLR 1151.

It has also been found that a healthcare practitioner cannot be held responsible for the consequences of a complication that they could not reasonably have been expected to anticipate (*see* Box 6.6).

BOX 6.6 The doctor is not responsible for unforeseeable complications[12]

In 1953, two patients sued an anaesthetist for negligence after they were left painfully crippled following surgery under spinal anaesthesia on the same operating list. It was believed that their painful debility was the result of the local anaesthetic solution becoming contaminated by phenol, the chemical used to sterilise the ampoules. The phenol was thought to have leached into the local anaesthetic through microscopic flaws in the glass. It was judged that the anaesthetist could not realistically have been expected to anticipate this problem, and he was found not liable.

Medical manslaughter

The sedationist must ensure that he or she is practising in a manner that would be acceptable to a responsible body of health professionals. Not to do so could lead not only to a claim of negligence, but also to a criminal charge of manslaughter if the patient subsequently died. To be charged with manslaughter after a medical accident, there must be causation, but in addition the practitioner's breach of duty must have been so blatant as to be regarded as reckless. This was clarified by the case of *R v Adomako* (*see* Box 6.7).

BOX 6.7 Reckless negligence

Dr A was an anaesthetist who took over the management of a patient undergoing eye surgery. Dr A accepted the case at 10.30, and at about 11.05 the breathing system delivering oxygen to the patient became detached from the endotracheal tube. Dr A did not become alert to the situation until some time later, when the patient developed low blood pressure and a bradycardia. Cardiac arrest resulted at 11.14. Dr A's care was described as 'abysmal' and 'a gross dereliction.' It was found that his negligence was 'reckless' to the extent that it met the criminal standard. He was convicted of manslaughter. This was confirmed on appeal.

R v Adomako [1994] 3 All ER 81.

The number of doctors prosecuted for manslaughter arising from the performance of their duties is small, but has risen steeply since the early 1990s. However, the conviction rate remains low. Most prosecutions arise from individual errors,[13–15] although some of the cases resulted from systems failures which left one or more individuals exposed to personal culpability. The questions that often need to be answered legally are whether the health practitioner made an error, whether they were solely responsible for that error, and whether the error can be divorced from the serious consequences that resulted in harm. The low conviction rates suggest that the criminal court is not the best forum for dealing with most of these cases, and the rising number of prosecutions may reflect a poor regulatory and legal framework with regard to a complex and challenging field of practice such as healthcare. The details of some prosecutions for medical manslaughter are shown in Boxes 6.8 and 6.9.[13–15]

BOX 6.8 Incorrect drug administered[14]

A doctor administered what he thought was diazepam to a patient who was undergoing a minor surgical procedure. The patient collapsed, and despite hospital treatment, died. It was subsequently found that the doctor had injected methohexitone – a barbiturate general anaesthetic – in error. Prosecution took place on the basis that the doctor was alleged to have attempted to provide anaesthesia alone and unaccompanied. The doctor was eventually acquitted.

BOX 6.9 Incorrect sedation technique

A GP performed circumcisions on young boys, utilising diamorphine as a sedative. A 9-year-old boy was subsequently found to have suffered brain damage. The doctor pleaded guilty to manslaughter, having given 'excessive amounts of these drugs, and it was accepted that they were wholly inappropriate as sedatives.' The doctor was sentenced to 12 months in prison, suspended for 12 months.

Doctor admits killing. *Guardian*, 4 March 1994.

The operator-sedationist

Although the anaesthetic fraternity quite rightly frowns upon the practice of *operator-anaesthetist*, the role of *operator-sedationist* is well established. In these circumstances, the operator provides the sedation, and then performs the operative procedure. There are several caveats to this practice. First, the patient, the environment and the technique used must all be suitable and safe, and must adhere to appropriate standards. Secondly, while performing the operative procedure, the operator quite clearly cannot observe the effects of the sedation on the patient, and must delegate that task to another appropriately trained individual. This individual must be able to understand how to monitor the patient properly and how to recognise important changes in observations, and must be able to intervene appropriately. The observer must therefore be able to act independently of the operator, as the operator may not be able to stop the procedure to assist if a problem arises. An observer who relies completely on the guidance of the operator-sedationist is not a suitable person to whom to delegate tasks of this type. Those who delegate a task to a person who is unable to provide the minimum standard of skill to perform that task are in breach of guidance from their regulatory bodies.

Sedation provided for a nurse-operator

Historically, the operator has been an appropriately trained doctor or dentist. However, more and more practitioners from other disciplines, particularly nurses, are able to perform medical procedures. Where a doctor is providing anaesthesia or sedation for another doctor or a dentist, the situation with regard to responsibility for the patient's well-being is clearly defined. The surgeon has responsibility for performing the surgery, and the anaesthetist/ sedationist is responsible for their own practice. With regard to a non-doctor providing sedation for a doctor, although the non-doctor is responsible for their own actions, the doctor still retains overall accountability for the patient's safety, and may be subject to disciplinary action if it is felt that they have delegated the task of sedation (or observation) to an inappropriate individual. However, it is not clear where the ultimate responsibility lies when a doctor is providing sedation for a nurse surgeon. This may not yet occur very often, if at all. However, the Royal College of Anaesthetists produced a statement covering this situation.[16] In essence, if the nurse surgeon is directly responsible within a defined framework to a named doctor, and practising with their approval, the medical anaesthetist/sedationist is not accountable for any error that they make. However, if the nurse surgeon is practising outside of such a clinical governance framework, the medical anaesthetist/ sedationist may be taken to have delegated care of the operation to the nurse, and may well be found responsible for any resulting error that the nurse may make. This has not yet been tested in law.

Documentation

It is a simple medico-legal maxim that if an event was not recorded in the patient's notes, it did not happen. If a practitioner sees a patient, or makes an intervention in their care, it is only sensible to ensure that this is documented appropriately. Such records should be dated and timed (including a note explaining any delay if they are not written soon after the consultation), and should be clearly attributable to the writer. They should be legible, truthful and as complete as possible. Given that there is always the possibility of a complaint of some kind, the author of the record should ensure that the note is detailed enough to allow them to justify their actions at a date far in the future.

A sedationist should therefore ensure that there is a record of the consent process for sedation, a record of any pre-operative assessment that was made, a record of the sedation and surgery, including the post-operative period, and a record of the discharge process.

It is important to remember that the data recorded by the observer-sedationist during the operative procedure may be the only contemporaneous record of events. As such, the observer-sedationist needs to record appropriate activities and observations on a time-based record. This will include drugs administered (including the use of oxygen), parameters derived from monitors, and relevant events (e.g. operation start time, time when a tourniquet was applied and removed, etc.) and interventions. It is certainly prudent to record that the level of sedation provided was checked at regular intervals.[17]

Regulatory framework

Healthcare professionals are responsible for their own actions, but may also be accountable for the actions of others (*see* Box 6.10).

BOX 6.10 A professional's accountability for the actions of others

A dental surgeon faced disciplinary action from the GDC following the death of a boy during sedation for routine dental surgery. The dentist did not appreciate his responsibilities for ensuring that the doctor providing sedation was using an appropriate technique.

Dentist fights for job after drugs blunder; www.cambridge-news.co.uk/news/city/2006/10/05/de7944b7-f263-46ff-926e-a (accessed 20 June 2007).

As a result, the sedationist may have to answer for their actions to their patients, the Law, their employers, and also the regulatory body that governs their professional activities. The General Medical Council (GMC), the General Dental Council (GDC) and the Nursing and Midwifery Council (NMC) are the most relevant professional bodies in this regard. They have responsibilities to maintain a register of qualified practitioners, to produce and maintain codes of practice, to investigate complaints, to take disciplinary action and to advise on education. The codes of conduct have several common threads, which are summarised in Table 6.1.[18–20] Significant breaches of the code of conduct may call into question an individual's fitness to practise.

TABLE 6.1 Common threads in the Codes of Conduct produced by the GMC, the GDC and the NMC

Make the care of the patient your first concern. This includes respecting their dignity, autonomy and confidentiality, and respecting their beliefs.

Keep your professional skills and knowledge up to date. Ensure that you practise within the limits of your competency at all times. This includes asking for more senior help when required.

Uphold the public trust in the profession by maintaining your integrity, and by being trustworthy and honest. This will include cooperating to resolve complaints.

Ensure that you are working well as part of a multi-disciplinary team. Treat your fellow professionals with respect.

Manage risks appropriately. This will include ensuring that patients are protected at all times. This may include reporting concerns about your own health and that of other professionals to the appropriate body.

Summary

The law surrounding healthcare practice is a specialist and complicated field that is developing all the time. Nevertheless, all healthcare professionals should be clear about what their professional, personal and legal responsibilities are, and ensure that they adhere to appropriate standards of practice at all times. It may be that their responsibilities are found to extend beyond the boundaries that they expected.

LEARNING POINTS

- Healthcare workers must be aware of the legal framework within which they practise.
- Sedationists must be satisfied that the patient has given informed consent for both the procedure and the sedation.
- The sedationist must be aware of the standard to which they are expected to practise.
- The legal and professional responsibilities of healthcare workers can be more extensive than they may have expected.

References

1 *Oxford Popular English Dictionary.* Oxford: Oxford University Press; 2001.

2 Department of Health. *Reference Guide to Consent for Examination and Treatment;* www.doh.gov.uk/consent (accessed 21 May 2007).

3 Adams S. *Good Practice in Consent. Achieving the NHS Plan commitment to patient-centred consent practice;* www.doh.gov.uk/publications/coinh.html (accessed 20 April 2007).

4 Lemaire F. The Nuremberg doctors' trial: the 60th anniversary. *Intensive Care Med.* 2006; **32:** 2049–52.

5 Vyvyan HAL, Hanafiah Z. Patients' attitudes to rectal drug administration. *Anaesthesia.* 1995; **50:** 983–4.

6 Mazur DJ. Influence of the law on risk and informed consent. *BMJ.* 2003; **327:** 731–4.

7 General Medical Council. *Withdrawing Life-Prolonging Treatments: good practice in decision making;* www.gmc-uk.org/guidance/current/library/witholding_lifeprolonging_guidance.asp (accessed 22 August 2007).

8 Association of Anaesthetists of Great Britain and Ireland. *Consent for Anaesthesia.* Revised ed; www.aagbi.org/publications/guidelines/docs/consent06.pdf (accessed 7 July 2007).

9 Royal College of Anaesthetists Patient Liaison Group. *Consent for Care or Treatment Given by an Anaesthetist;* www.rcoa.ac.uk/docs/Consent_june05.pdf (accessed 12 April 2007).

10 White SM, Baldwin TJ. Consent for anaesthesia. *Anaesthesia.* 2003; **58:** 760–74.

11 UK Academy of Medical Royal Colleges and their Faculties. *Implementing and Ensuring Safe Sedation Practice for Healthcare Procedures in Adults. Report of an Intercollegiate Working Group, Royal College of Anaesthetists;* www.rcoa.ac.uk/docs/safesedationpractice.pdf (accessed 17 August 2007).

12 Hutter CD. The Wooley and Roe case. A reassessment. *Anaesthesia.* 1990; **45:** 859–64.

13 Holbrook J. The criminalisation of fatal medical mistakes. *BMJ.* 2003; **327:** 1118–19.

14 Ferner RE. Medication errors that have led to manslaughter charges. *BMJ.* 2000; **321:** 1212–16.

15 Ferner RE, McDowell SE. Doctors charged with manslaughter in the course of medical practice, 1795–2005: a literature review. *J R Soc Med.* 2006; **99:** 309–14.

16 Royal College of Anaesthetists. Interim position statement on the provision of anaesthetic services for procedures performed by non-medically qualified operators; www.rcoa.ac.uk/printindex.asp?PageID=702 (accessed 12 April 2007).

17 Royal College of Anaesthetists, Association of Anaesthetists of Great Britain and Ireland, and the Society for Computing and Technology in Anaesthesia. *Anaesthetic Record Set.* London: Royal College of Anaesthetists, Association of Anaesthetists of Great Britain and Ireland, and the Society for Computing and Technology in Anaesthesia; 1996.

18 General Dental Council. *The Principles of Practice in Dentistry;* www.gdc-uk. org/NR/rdonlyres/23636B75-1E3F-463E-930E-9E21EAF72141/17062/147158_ Standards_Profs.pdf (accessed 25 May 2007).

19 General Medical Council. *Good Medical Practice;* www.gmc-uk.org/guidance/ good_medical_practice/how_gmp_applies_to_you.asp (accessed 7 July 2007).

20 Nursing and Midwifery Council. *The NMC Code of Professional Conduct: standards for conduct, performance and ethics;* www.nmc-uk.org/aDisplayDocument. aspx?DocumentID=201 (accessed 22 August 2007).

Further reading

Landmark legal cases

Bolam v Friern Hospital Management Committee [1957] 1 WLR 582.

Bolitho v City and Hackney Health Authority [1997] 3 WLR 1151.

Chester v Afshar [2004] UKHL 41.

Gillick v West Norfolk and Wisbech Health Authority [1985] 3 All ER 402.

Salgo v Leland Stanford Junior University Board of Trustees [1957] 317 P.2d 170 (Cal. Dist. Ct. App. 1957).

Sidaway v Bethlehem Royal Hospital [1985] AL 871 HL.

Wilsher v Essex Health Authority [1986] 3 All ER 801.

Relevant medico-legal textbooks

Campbell B, Callum K, Peacock NA. *Operating Within the Law. A practical guide for surgeons and lawyers.* Shrewsbury: TFM Publishing; 2001.

Davies M. *Textbook on Medical Law.* 2nd ed. Oxford: Blackstone Press; 1998.

Hambly PR. *Essential Reports for Anaesthetists.* Oxford: Bios Publishing; 1997.

Marquand P. *Introduction to Medical Law.* Oxford: Butterworth-Heinemann; 2000.

CHAPTER 7

Sedation in paediatric practice

Children may require sedation for procedures which in an adult one might expect to be achieved solely with reassurance. However, children can react unpredictably at times of stress, resulting in behaviour which renders the proposed procedure impossible. Alternatively, they may be unable to keep still for the duration of the procedure without sedation. It is also usual in most cases that a parent, carer or guardian accompanies the child during part or all of the sedation process and/or the procedure. The sedationist will therefore have to utilise their skills to reassure both the patient and the parent/carer. It must be noted that much work in this area has been done in the USA, where it is acknowledged that 'deep sedation is required for most procedures.'[1] As deep sedation is regarded as a level of anaesthesia in the UK, many of these suggested North American techniques are not directly applicable to UK practice.

Although the principles of safe sedation practice for children will be the same as those for adults, the knowledge base and skills required by the sedationist are substantially different. Sedation for children does require many specific considerations, including familiarity with specialist equipment and paediatric physiology.

Paediatric practice encompasses a wide range of patients, varying in size, age, physiology and anatomy. As a general rule, the post-pubertal child can be treated as if they were a 'small-scale adult' in terms of physiology and pharmacology. However, the younger the child, the greater is the deviation from the adult condition. Although the sedationist should always be alert for potential hazards, it is clear that the scope for problems arising in children is much greater than that in adults. It is recommended that sedation is only administered to paediatric patients by those for whom this is regular practice.

For the purposes of this chapter, the following terms are used:

➧ **premature baby:** a baby born before full gestation (38–40 weeks) has been completed

➧ **neonate:** any child less than 4 weeks old (within 44 weeks of conceptual age)

➧ **infant:** a child older than 4 weeks, but within the first year of life

➧ **child:** a child older than 1 year who is pre-pubertal

➧ **adolescent:** a post-pubertal child

➧ **children:** a generic term encompassing all of the above.

General principles of paediatric sedation

Complication rates for sedation in children have been quoted by various studies as ranging from 1.2% to 2.3% where single agents are used, but have been noted to increase markedly when techniques that utilise multiple drugs are implemented. Coté[2] and his colleagues reviewed 118 reported adverse events related to paediatric sedation from a variety of American databases. In total, 95 of these events were suitable for analysis, of which 60 had resulted in death or poor neurological outcome. There was no relationship between events and the type of sedation drug utilised, or route of administration. However, adverse events were often associated with an excessive dose. Events were more common with combinations of drugs, poor choice of technique, human errors, lack of skills or lack of monitoring. It was notable that a proportion of the sedation-related events occurred in the recovery period rather than during the procedure. One recorded death, associated with the use of chloral hydrate, occurred while the child was on the way to hospital in their parent's car, the sedative having been given as a premedication at home. Other research has reported a higher incidence of adverse events.[3]

Paediatric sedation practice was subjected to a rigorous review by the Scottish Intercollegiate Guidelines Network (SIGN) in 2004.[4] The main recommendations arising from this report, which are summarised in Table 7.1, are supported by other international publications.[5]

The SIGN document was subject to some criticism[6] with regard to the quoted evidence used to support some of the recommendations. However, the document is recognised as a basic guide to safe practice, and its recommendations remain a key governance consideration.

TABLE 7.1 Summary of the SIGN 58 recommendations[4]

Principles of good practice	■ An individualised approach is required in order to minimise fear, anxiety, pain and distress, while at the same time allowing the procedure to be accomplished safely, reliably and efficiently, whilst respecting the rights of the child. ■ Consent should be obtained prior to the procedure, and should include a full description of the sedation to be employed. The possibility of failure and later general anaesthetic should be discussed. This should normally be undertaken and recorded by the sedationist. ■ Gentle, protective containment and positioning are permitted, but forcible restraint is not. Every institution should possess a guideline as to what is and is not allowable, and staff should be regularly trained in these methods. If the child is uncooperative, the best option may be to abandon the procedure and re-list them for a general anaesthetic. ■ Parental involvement may have a sedative-sparing effect.
Environmental considerations	■ Sedation should only be performed in an environment where the facilities, personnel and equipment necessary to manage paediatric emergency situations are immediately available. ■ Sedation should occur as near as possible to the area where the procedure is to be performed. Transfer of sedated children should only be undertaken by appropriately trained and skilled staff. ■ Facilities that must be available are similar to those required for general anaesthesia, and include oxygen, emergency airway equipment, resuscitation equipment, suction and appropriate monitors.
Personnel	■ The sedationist should be trained to provide at least basic paediatric life support. Training in advanced paediatric life support is encouraged. ■ Although the roles of the operator and the sedationist may overlap, the operator should not be the person responsible for monitoring the child during the procedure. ■ The sedationist must be able to manage the patient if a deeper level of sedation than intended is achieved. ■ Nurse sedation services may be appropriate in some environments. These nurse practitioners would be expected to have the skills required of any sedationist.

cont.

Patients	■ Patients should be subject to a proper pre-procedure assessment to ensure that no contraindications to sedation are present.
	■ Only ASA grade 1 and 2 patients should be considered for outpatient sedation (and possibly ASA 3 with stable illness in some circumstances).
	■ Pre-operative preparation should include behavioural techniques.
	■ The child should be subject to fasting as with a general anaesthetic (this requirement may be varied if nitrous oxide is the only agent being used).

General considerations in paediatric sedation practice

Pre-operative period

Consent is not a straightforward issue in children. Briefly, below the age of majority, children are assumed to lack the capacity to consent to treatment, and consent is therefore taken from the child's parents or guardian. However, some children might be judged to have capacity, and so will be able to consent to treatment in the absence of a responsible adult. It is for the health professionals to decide whether the child has such capacity. If the parents refuse consent, then the health professionals may have to obtain a court order to allow treatment. However, in an emergency, treatment can be given without consent if it is judged by the health practitioners that the intervention is in the patient's best interests. Written informed consent for sedation should be obtained and recorded, preferably by the practitioner who is providing the sedation. This should include information about the proposed technique and the alternatives available. It should include the fact that if sedation fails, a general anaesthetic at a later date may be necessary.

Although the range of illnesses that affect children may be broadly the same as those in adults, there are also conditions, particularly those with a genetic origin, which can be unique to childhood. Many of these conditions can be associated with airway abnormalities, as well as with abnormalities in other organs. Heart defects occur in approximately 7 cases per 1000 live births, 10% of which will also be linked with non-cardiac problems.

Children should be carefully selected for sedation, and consideration given to performing the procedure under an anaesthetic if there is any doubt about safety. Children with long-term illnesses (e.g. cancer) may be subject to multiple procedures, and in these cases it may be more suitable to consider a general anaesthetic from the outset, in order to minimise psychological trauma. Both parents and child should be aware that if sedation is unsuccessful, the safest option may be to abandon the procedure and arrange for a general anaesthetic at a later date, rather than to persist and deepen sedation to an anaesthetic level. This is particularly true in circumstances where the child has had paradoxical agitation with midazolam.[7] During pre-procedure assessment, any contraindications to sedation should be actively sought. These will need to be dealt with appropriately before sedation can take place, or the procedure will have to be abandoned. Common contraindications are listed in Table 7.2.

TABLE 7.2 Common contraindications to sedation

CONTRAINDICATION	REASON
Abnormal airway	Risk of obstruction and hypoxia
Raised intracranial pressure	Respiratory depression, leading to raised carbon dioxide level, and further pressure increases
Sleep apnoea	Risk of airway depression with sedatives and opiates
Respiratory failure, cardiac failure	Risk of deterioration during procedure
Neuromuscular disease	Reduced respiratory reserve and increased risk of respiratory depression
Bowel obstruction	Aspiration
Active respiratory tract infection	Post-procedure chest infection
Known allergy to proposed drugs/ adverse reaction	Anaphylaxis
Child distressed and/or uncooperative	May result in inability to perform the procedure, or injury
Consent refused	Advice would need to be taken as to how to proceed

Exactly the same principles apply to the selection of paediatric patients as for adult patients. Children should be assessed and classified according to ASA criteria. As a general principle, ASA grade 1 and 2 children are probably suitable for sedation. Selected ASA grade 3 children in certain circumstances may also be suitable, depending upon the environment, resources and proposed procedure. Some authorities have suggested that children should be scored an ASA grade 'higher' than the corresponding 'adult' grade, to remind staff of the different hazards involved.

Behavioural therapy techniques may reduce the requirement for sedation. The use of *play therapy* and so-called 'Saturday Clubs' (where children attending for a procedure can come to the hospital the weekend before admission in order to become familiarised with the ward) can be very helpful in this regard. *Distraction therapy* can be extremely useful for quick, painful procedures (e.g. blood sampling). However, in some cases careful planning may obviate the need for sedation altogether. For example, for a painless procedure (e.g. X-ray imaging), sleep deprivation for a period before the test may be sufficient to ensure the cooperation of the child. Feeding an infant may lead to postprandial drowsiness sufficient to allow a procedure to be performed without pharmacological intervention. If a child is particularly anxious, sedative premedication can be given the evening before.

Pre-procedure fasting may be as necessary for sedation as it is for anaesthesia in order to minimise the risk of aspiration. Smaller children cannot tolerate periods of fasting as well as older children or adults. A variety of recommendations have been made with regard to this issue, and the sedationist should ensure that they are aware of the recommendations in use at their institute. Typical guidance is shown in Table 7.3. This means that the timing of sedation and procedures in relation to fasting times is an important consideration.

TABLE 7.3 An example of anaesthetic paediatric pre-procedure fasting guidelines

TYPE OF FLUID	TIME OF FASTING
Clear fluid	2 hours
Breast milk	4 hours
Formula milk	4–6 hours
Food	6 hours

A clear fluid is one that does not contain milk, and through which newspaper print can be easily read. This does not include carbonated drinks.

It is recommended that children who are likely to have complex sedation requirements are treated only within an environment that meets the standards required to provide general anaesthesia. In these cases, an appropriately trained anaesthetist should be the sedationist.

Considerations during sedation

The sedation technique that is utilised should be tried and tested, and performed in accordance with local guidelines. The procedures that are adopted can be based upon national guidelines, or those of specialist centres. The guidelines for Great Ormond Street Hospital are currently available at www.ich.ucl.ac.uk/clinserv/anaesthetics/professionals/03sedation.html

Drug doses in children are calculated on a 'mg per kg' basis. This means that all children will need to be weighed. Failing this, their weight can be estimated from various formulae (*see* Table 7.4). Alternatively, use can be made of specific tools, such as the Walsall Paediatric Resuscitation Chart, which gives guidance on weight, drug doses and endotracheal tube size for children, based on the age of the child. Incorrect calculation of drug dosage can have catastrophic consequences (*see* Box 7.1).

TABLE 7.4 Formulae for estimating approximate weight

CHILD'S AGE		APPROXIMATE WEIGHT FORMULA	EXAMPLE
Less than 12 months old		[Age (months) + 9]/2	A 9-month-old child will weigh approximately 9 kg
More than 12 months old		[Age (years) + 4] × 2	A 4-year-old child can be assumed to weigh approximately 16 kg
Age (years)	Approximate weight (kg)		
Full term	3.5		
Neonate	4.2		
3 months	6		
6 months	7.5		
1 year	10		
5 years	18		
10	30		

BOX 7.1 Miscalculated paediatric drug dose

L, a premature, 7-day-old child, developed breathing difficulties on a Neonatal Intensive-Care Unit. It was determined by the consultant, Dr S, that a chest drain was required. As pain relief would be needed, Dr S asked for the child to be given morphine before the procedure. Dr M, the registrar, administered a dose of morphine that had been prepared by Dr E, the SHO. Unfortunately, Dr E had miscalculated the dosage, and L received *100 times* the intended amount. Despite treatment, she subsequently died. At the inquest, Dr E's mistake in converting a dose from 'micrograms' to 'milligrams' was described as 'damn silly and reckless.' It was revealed that a previous incident involving a baby receiving *10 times* the proper dose of morphine had occurred on the same unit 2 months before. A verdict of accidental death was returned. All three doctors were found not guilty of serious professional misconduct by the General Medical Council.

GMC investigates baby drug death (24 July 1998); http://news.bbc.co.uk/1/hi/health/

Overdose doctor cleared (20 April 1999); http://news.bbc.co.uk/1/hi/health/138612.stm

Doctor thought overdose was safe (21 April 1999); http://news.bbc.co.uk/1/hi/health/325228.stm

Overdose doctors cleared (23 April 1999); http://news.bbc.co.uk/1/hi/health/326656.stm
(All websites accessed 18 April 2007)

Successful use of sedation will depend on the skill and judgement of the sedationist and their relationship with the child and his or her parents/guardian. The parents may be allowed to accompany the child, but should be carefully briefed as to what to expect, and as to how they may be asked to assist. Parental presence may obviate the need for sedation, and is certainly sedative sparing in most cases. However, attendance should not be compulsory, as an agitated parent may well increase the distress of a child.[8] The staff who are caring for the child should also be made aware of any suspicions about the nature of the child–parent relationship.[9]

It may be difficult to distinguish between sedation and anaesthesia in children because of age and/or verbal communication issues, or because the procedure prevents verbalisation. In these cases, other means of communication should be established (e.g. 'thumbs up', 'thumbs down', hand squeezing, etc.). If communication with the child is lost because of sedation, the standard of care provided needs to be the same as that required for anaesthesia. A variety of specific paediatric sedation scales have been developed for use by clinicians. The Wilton sedation scale[10] is reproduced in Table 7.5.

TABLE 7.5 An example of a paediatric sedation scale: the Wilton sedation scale

Agitated	Clinging to parent, crying
Alert	Awake, not clinging, not crying
Calm	Sitting/lying comfortably with eyes open
Drowsy	Sitting/lying comfortably with eyes spontaneously closing, but responding to minor stimulation
Asleep	Eyes closed, rousable, but does not respond to minor stimulation

Hypoventilation, laryngospasm and airway obstruction are particular airway risks, which can be minimised – but not totally eliminated – by careful assessment and preparation.[4,11,12]

Anatomy and physiology

Paediatric anatomy and physiology can differ markedly from the adult equivalent. Some paediatric parameters are shown in Table 7.6. In order to practise safely, the sedationist needs a good understanding of childhood physiology, and how it can change depending upon the age of the child.

TABLE 7.6 Paediatric physiological parameters

AGE (YEARS)	PULSE RATE (BEATS/MINUTE)	MEAN SYSTOLIC BLOOD PRESSURE (MMHG)	AVERAGE BLOOD VOLUME (ML/KG)
Neonate	80–200	50–90	90
1	80–160	85–105	85
5	80–120	95–110	80
10	70–110	100–120	
12	60–110	110–130	

Airway and breathing

The airway of a young child is more difficult to manage during anaesthesia and resuscitation than that of an older child or an adult. For example, in infants the tongue is relatively larger and the mouth is relatively smaller than in older children. The face can be chubby, so specially shaped face masks may be required to support ventilation during anaesthesia. The adoption of the traditional 'sniffing the morning air' position for mask ventilation may obstruct, rather than optimise, the airway of the neonate or infant, so the 'head neutral' position is preferred in this age group. The epiglottis is larger, and may obstruct the view of the larynx if endotracheal intubation is needed.

As a result, paediatric emergency airway equipment is not just a scaled down version of adult equipment. Round rather than 'anatomical' face masks are used for infants, as they contain less respiratory 'dead space', straight rather than curved laryngoscope blades may be required, and so on.

Any area in which children are sedated will need to possess, or have rapid access to, appropriate paediatric equipment. The sedationist should ensure that this equipment is available and that it has been checked.

Premature babies, neonates and infants

The physiology of such children is significantly different to that of the older child. Oxygenation is dependent mainly on respiratory rate, which may be about twice that of a normal adult. Poorly developed thoracic musculature in neonates and premature babies means that respiratory fatigue is more common under conditions of stress, so apnoea can be a significant post-procedure problem. Lung alveoli may still be developing, so gas exchange can be less efficient. A neonate will have a large proportion of fetal haemoglobin as opposed to normal adult haemoglobin, which means that a pulse oximeter may read high or normal saturations at relatively low circulating oxygen levels. The higher metabolic rate means that the neonate and infant have higher oxygen consumption, and so will desaturate and become cyanosed alarmingly quickly. Similarly, the cardiac output is rate dependent, so bradycardia is an alarming sign which must be treated aggressively. In association with hypoxia, a slow heart rate can be regarded as pre-terminal. Venous access can be very difficult due to small vein diameter, chubby hands and a lack of cooperation. The blood volume of a neonate is proportionally larger than that of an infant or a child (*see* Table 7.6), although the overall volume is smaller. Deceptively small amounts of blood loss can lead to circulatory compromise. The functions of the liver and the kidney are not mature, so the handling of drugs can be unpredictable. As a result of their immature metabolism, neonates and infants can become hypoglycaemic very quickly. The surface area of the neonate and the infant is relatively large compared with their volume, so they can lose heat very rapidly. Appropriate measures, such as warming the room in which the procedure is to take place, and covering the scalp, should be utilised.

Resuscitation

Both the sedationist and the team managing the child will need to be proficient in the resuscitation techniques utilised in children of different ages. Many courses that provide training in paediatric resuscitation are available. The Advanced Paediatric Life Support (APLS) course is extremely detailed and thorough, and is based on established guidelines.[13] APLS providers must ensure that their skills are regularly revalidated. Resuscitation protocols are updated frequently, and staff must ensure that these alterations in practice are properly disseminated. The current guidelines will be available from national resuscitation organisations and their websites (details of the Resuscitation Council in the UK can be found at www.resus.org.uk).

As in adults, the paediatric resuscitation guideline follows an 'ABC' (Airway, Breathing, Circulation) framework. However, it differs significantly in that the commonest cause of cardiac arrest in adults is heart disease, whereas cardiac arrest in children (without congenital heart disease) is usually the result of hypoxia, and therefore the outcome is very likely to be death. Respiratory problems are common complications during sedation, so the sedationist should be extremely vigilant in monitoring the patency of the paediatric airway, and must be prepared to deal with any emergency that arises. Any signs of respiratory insufficiency in the sedated child must be taken extremely seriously. The airway is of primary concern, so those involved in the sedation of children must be able to anticipate difficulty, recognise an inadequate airway, and be able to take remedial action while summoning expert anaesthetic or paediatric help. If there are signs of impending airway difficulty (e.g. noisy breathing), simple airway manipulation such as optimising the head position and opening the mouth may be all that is required. This can be achieved with the chin lift or jaw thrust manoeuvre, which pull the tongue away from the back of the pharynx. It is important to remember that if the child is not responsive, they are either anaesthetised or collapsed.

TABLE 7.7 **Summary of current basic and advanced life support**

BASIC PAEDIATRIC LIFE SUPPORT	ADVANCED PAEDIATRIC LIFE SUPPORT
Is the child unresponsive? Shout for help.	Basic life support commenced. Help is on the way.
Open the airway. Is the child breathing? If Yes, support the airway and give oxygen. If No, give five rescue breaths.	Attach cardiac monitor and assess rhythm. Is the rhythm shockable (ventricular fibrillation/ pulseless ventricular tachycardia) or not shockable (pulseless electrical activity/asystole)?
Is the circulation adequate? If No, commence CPR.	If the rhythm is shockable: Deliver defibrillatory shock. Recommence CPR for 2 minutes. Reassess rhythm. Shock again if necessary. Continue until rhythm changes/child recovers/child dies.
Institute advanced life support, or continue basic life support until help arrives.	If the rhythm is not shockable: Continue CPR. Check rhythm and pulse every 2 minutes. Continue until rhythm changes/child recovers/child dies.

Remember to look for reversible causes (e.g. hypoxia, hyper- or hypokalaemia, hypothermia, hypovolaemia, tension pneumothorax, cardiac tamponade, thromboembolism, drug-related problems, etc.).

The adequacy of the airway can be checked by looking for chest movement, listening for air flow or abnormal sounds, and placing the head next to the patient's mouth to feel the air flow on the cheek. This should take no more than 10 seconds. If the airway is not adequate, the rescuer will need to administer up to five breaths via a bag and mask attached to high-flow oxygen, two of which should be seen to cause chest movement. Once this has occurred, the rescuer needs to check the adequacy of the circulation. An absent central pulse, or the presence of bradycardia, should lead to commencement of cardiac compressions alternating with ventilation in a ratio of 15 chest compressions to every two breaths at a rate of 100 compressions a minute. This is summarised in Table 7.7.

Life support should continue until the child's condition improves or skilled help arrives. In the mean time, consideration should be given to any reversible causes of arrest which could be easily treatable (e.g. pneumothorax). Defibrillation may be necessary if the patient has developed ventricular fibrillation or pulseless ventricular tachycardia.

It is recommended that all of those involved in paediatric sedation should be trained in paediatric basic life support at the very least, and that an advanced paediatric life support provider is easily available. This is even more important in isolated clinics, where skilled paediatric and anaesthetic help may be some distance away, than it is in hospitals (*see* Box 7.2).

BOX 7.2 Staff not familiar with paediatric life support techniques

A consultant anaesthetist was struck off the medical register following the death of K, a 5-year-old girl, at a dental surgery. K had undergone anaesthesia for dental extractions, but had developed an obstructed airway. This went unnoticed because Dr V, the anaesthetist, had not utilised appropriate monitoring. It was also determined that Dr V had little knowledge relating to life support techniques – his approach to the resuscitation of K was described as 'shambolic.' During the resuscitation, an inappropriately high level of shock was administered. Dr V was found not guilty of manslaughter.

Dangerous doctor struck off (25 July 2002); http://news.bbc.co.uk/1/hi/england/2151196.stm (accessed 18 April 2007).

Other considerations

It is also expected that all staff involved in paediatric practice will be fully aware of their responsibilities with regard to child protection. This will include taking appropriate action if there are legitimate concerns, such as the presence of unexplained injury.[14–17]

Pharmacology of paediatric sedation[18]

Intravenous sedation

Midazolam is the most commonly used agent in this regard. Propofol, ketamine and barbiturates should only be used by anaesthetists in an appropriate environment. If intravenous sedation is to be used, it is recommended that a proper intravenous cannula rather than a 'butterfly'-type needle is in place.

Non-intravenous sedation

As intravascular access may be difficult, and intramuscular injection is quite painful (and tends to be avoided in paediatric practice unless there is good reason), other routes of drug administration in children have also been explored. This may be particularly useful when the aim is to produce a cooperative child by inducing anxiolysis for minor, non-painful procedures. It must be remembered that the effects of medication administered by a non-intravenous route may be unreliable, as the drug dose cannot be titrated to effect, and absorption through mucous membranes can be unpredictable. Onset of action may be delayed, and the duration of action may be prolonged.

The intravenous formulation of midazolam has been used for oral administration. Midazolam is quite bitter, and may need to be administered in a sweet-tasting drink. Paracetamol syrup in an appropriate dose has been used successfully in this context, and has the advantage of providing concomitant analgesia. Administration of oral sedative is more successful if it is given by syringe rather than by spoon. The dose is approximately 0.5 mg/kg, up to a maximum of 20 mg.

Nasal administration of midazolam has also been proposed, but is poorly tolerated and sometimes painful due to the irritant, acidic nature of the solution. However, specific formulations of nasal midazolam are available from selected sources. For example, a solution of 40 mg midazolam with 20 mg/ml of lidocaine is available on a named consultant basis (but not commercially). Supplied as a 0.5-ml ampoule (containing 20 mg of midazolam and 10 mg of lidocaine), it can be sprayed through an atomiser into the child's nasal passage. This 0.5-ml dose is suitable for use in children who weigh 25 kg or more. The dosage received is unpredictable, as the child may expel some of the solution (by sneezing, etc.), but the solution can reliably induce conscious sedation within about 15 minutes (W Hamlin, 2007, personal communication). The dose is usually quoted as 0.2 mg/kg.

The rectal route has also been used, but may not be acceptable culturally or individually, and will require specific consent.

Antihistamines have also been used, as they are known to have a sedative effect, although again it is unpredictable in nature. *Alimemazine* (*Vallergan*) is utilised in this manner, but is not licensed for use as a sedative in children under 2 years of age. *Trimeprazine* has been used, but is associated with hypotension. Combinations utilising agents such as *promethazine* and *pethidine* together have been given intramuscularly, but are associated with apnoea.

Chloral hydrate can also be given orally. It is metabolised to trichloroethanol in the bloodstream. It can cause gastric irritation and low blood pressure. It is extremely effective, but has been associated with respiratory depression and cardiac arrhythmia. It can have a prolonged effect, and it has been suggested that 89% of children have not returned to baseline activity by 24 hours after administration.[12] It is not licensed for the provision of sedation for painless procedures. It has been suggested that if chloral hydrate is used in combination with nitrous oxide, up to 94% of patients could be subject to deep sedation (i.e. anaesthesia).[19] *Triclofos* is similar to chloral hydrate, but causes fewer gastrointestinal side-effects. 1 mg of triclofos is equivalent to about 600 mg of chloral hydrate.

Other medications that have been given orally with success include *quinalbarbitone* and *melatonin*.

Ketamine has also been recommended by some authorities for use in children. It can be given intravenously, intramuscularly or orally. Although its analgesic properties may be of great use, they may be outweighed by its tendency to cause emergence hallucinations. It has been recommended that ketamine is used in combination with other agents such as midazolam in order to counter these effects.[20] It is suggested that ketamine does not tend to cause respiratory depression. However, this does not mean that the airway is not at risk at all, as this drug is associated with apnoea and laryngospasm.[21,22]

Nitrous oxide has also been used for sedation in children. Its rapid onset and offset and its analgesic properties are very useful. However, cooperation is required.

Some of these paediatric sedative medications are summarised in Table 7.8.

TABLE 7.8 Some commonly used paediatric sedative drugs

SEDATIVE	ADMINISTRATION ROUTE	DOSAGE	ONSET
Midazolam	Oral	0.5 mg/kg	20 minutes
	Nasal	0.2–0.5 mg/kg	20 minutes
	Intravenous	0.1 mg/kg	Minutes
Diazepam	Oral	1 month to 12 years, 200–300 mcg/kg (maximum 5 mg)	Variable
		12 to 18 years, 100–200 mcg/kg (maximum 20 mg)	
	Intravenous	1 month to 18 years, 100–220 mcg/kg over 4 minutes	Minutes
Alimemazine (Vallergan)	Oral	2 years to 7 years, 2 mg/kg (maximum 60 mg)	1–2 hours
Chloral hydrate	Oral	1 month to 12 years, 30–50 mg/kg (maximum 1 g)	45–60 minutes
		Over 12 years, 1–2 g	
Triclofos	Oral	1 month to 18 years, 30–50 mg/kg	60 minutes

The child should be closely monitored from the moment sedation has been administered. It should be remembered that paradoxical agitation can result from the use of any form of sedation, and will often require that the procedure is abandoned.

Specific procedures in paediatric practice

Children may have to undergo a variety of invasive or uncomfortable interventions or investigations. The level of sedation required will often depend upon whether the proposed procedure is painful or not, and the degree of cooperation required. Specific considerations with regard to some common procedures are summarised below.

Cardiology

Success in non-painful imaging procedures, such as echocardiography, is defined by the quality of the images produced, and therefore the cooperation of the child is paramount. Non-pharmacological methods such as sleep deprivation or performing the procedure after feeds may be successful in smaller children. In children over the age of 5 years, oral sedation may be required as an adjunct. Chloral hydrate, triclofos and midazolam have been found to be useful in this context. General anaesthesia is recommended for prolonged, uncomfortable procedures, such as trans-oesophageal echocardiography and cardiac catheterisation.

Casualty Department and minor procedures (e.g. wound care, drain removal, etc.)

Many procedures may be successfully performed by utilising reassurance, distraction therapy and play therapy, in combination with topical, infiltrated or regional anaesthesia, or in association with inhaled nitrous oxide. Nitrous oxide should only be utilised if the practitioner is familiar with the equipment that is being used to administer it. Opioids may be required for painful procedures, and can be given orally, nasally or intravenously. Midazolam can also be useful in these circumstances. It is not recommended that fentanyl, sufentanil, alfentanil, remifentanil, propofol, ketamine or other anaesthetic agents are used by non-anaesthetists in this environment. Fasting guidelines should normally apply.

Dentistry

This is covered in more detail in Chapter 9. An effort should be made to persuade the child to have simple dental procedures performed without sedation under local anaesthesia. Inhalational techniques utilising nitrous oxide are acceptable, but the equipment used must be appropriate and comply with safety standards. Inhalational sedation should be titrated to the patient's needs like any other method of sedation. It should only be undertaken using a dedicated relative analgesia machine that conforms to British Standards, and a waste gas scavenging system should be in place. Intravenous sedation with midazolam is only recommended in children over 16 years of age, and should be avoided in younger children in the primary care or community dental practice. It may be used in a specialist centre by a consultant-led team with appropriate expertise.

Gastrointestinal endoscopy

Single-drug sedation is unlikely to prove adequate, as it is necessary for the gag reflex to be suppressed for gastroscopy, and children are likely to react badly to the introduction of a colonoscope. For this reason, general anaesthesia is suggested as the best option for performing endoscopy in children. The sedationist should be aware that a large gastroscope could compress the airway of a small child.

Oncology

Children who are unfortunate enough to be suffering from cancer may be subjected to repeated invasive procedures or therapy. It may be possible to utilise behavioural techniques in combination with local anaesthesia for non-painful or brief procedures. However, it may be that a general anaesthetic is less psychologically damaging for a child who is subject to recurrent treatments.

Nephrology

General anaesthesia is the method of choice for renal biopsy and other similar procedures, due to the need for careful positioning and cooperation.

Neurology

Minor procedures such as lumbar puncture and intrathecal injections are usually possible under sedation, but a large number of children may require general anaesthesia.

Tests such as electroencephalograms (EEGs) and brainstem evoked potential (BSEP) may be difficult to interpret if sedation is used. For this reason, sleep deprivation or general anaesthesia is preferred, although melatonin has also been utilised.

Radiology

Procedures such as CT scanning and MRI imaging may be painless, but require cooperation. In addition, the child may be inside the device for a long period of time (e.g. for MRI spinal imaging). Good behavioural preparation may obviate the need for sedation in many cases. However, venous access should be obtained. Children less than 4 months old may be imaged without sedation when asleep, or after feeding.

Children who weigh less than 10 kg may be successfully sedated with a single dose of oral sedative, without significant risk of respiratory depression, although oral midazolam may be associated with a high risk of patient movement. The sedation should be given immediately prior to the procedure, and the sedationist should stay to observe the child. MRI scanning will require the use of non-ferromagnetic specialist monitoring equipment.

There is much debate in the anaesthetic world about the safety of sedation versus anaesthesia for MRI imaging in children.[23] What is certain is that some facilities have established perfectly safe and efficient paediatric sedation services for MRI scanning.[24–26] However, these successful services have developed as a result of close supervision and participation by the local anaesthetic department.

Painful radiological procedures, such as biopsy, drainage and dilatation, are probably best performed under an anaesthetic in children.

Summary

The principles of safe sedation for children are the same as those used in adult practice. However, a specific supplemental knowledge and skill base is required, as anatomy and physiology can differ significantly between children. Paediatric practice should not be approached in a casual manner. Sedationists should check the dose of medication that they plan to use with a reputable source, such as local guidelines or the *British National Formulary for Children*.[27]

LEARNING POINTS

- Anatomy and physiology can vary between different children, and can differ significantly from the adult equivalent.
- The sedation team should be specifically trained to deal with children, and all members of the team should be trained in paediatric life support.
- Hypoxia is a particular hazard in paediatric practice.
- Cardiac arrest in children is often the result of hypoxia, so survivability is low.
- Specific paediatric equipment must be available.

References

1 Hertzog JH, Havidich JE. Non-anaesthesiologist-provided paediatric procedural sedation: an update. *Curr Opin Anaesthesiol.* 2007; **20:** 365–72.

2 Coté CJ, Karl HW, Notterman DA *et al.* Adverse sedation events in pediatrics: analysis of medications used for sedation. *Pediatrics.* 2000; **106:** 633–44.

3 Malviya S, Voepal-Lewis T, Tait AR. Adverse events and risk factors associated with the sedation of children by non-anaesthetists. *Anesth Analg.* 1997; **85:** 1207–13.

4 Scottish Intercollegiate Guidelines Network. *SIGN 58: safe sedation in children undergoing diagnostic and therapeutic procedures. A national clinical guideline;* www.sign.ac.uk (accessed 11 March 2007).

5 Coté CJ, Wilson S and the Working Group on Sedation. *Guidelines for Monitoring and Management of Pediatric Patients During and After Sedation for Diagnostic and Therapeutic Procedures: an update;* www.pediatrics.org/cgi/content/full/118/6/2587 (accessed 13 May 2007).

6 Royal College of Paediatrics and Child Health Quality of Practice Committee. *Guideline Appraisal. Scottish Intercollegiate Guidelines Network (SIGN) evidence-based guidelines for the safe sedation of children undergoing diagnostic and therapeutic procedures*; www.rcpch.ac.uk/publications/clinical_docs/safe_sedation%20.pdf (accessed 13 May 2007).

7 Massanari M, Novitsky J, Reinstein LJ. Paradoxical reactions in children associated with midazolam use during endoscopy. *Clin Pediatr.* 1997; **36:** 681–4.

8 Seddon S. Should parents accompany children to the anaesthetic room? *Midlands Med.* 1994; **19:** 116–17.

9 Watts J. Parental presence during the induction of anaesthesia. *Anaesthesia.* 1997; **52:** 276–90.

10 Wilton NCT, Leigh J, Rosen DR *et al.* Pre-anaesthetic sedation of preschool children using intranasal midazolam. *Anaesthesiology.* 1988; **69:** 972–5.

11 Coté CJ, Alderfer RJ, Nottermann DA *et al.* Sedation disasters: adverse drug reports in pediatrics. *Anaesthesiology.* 1995: **83:** A1183.

12 Blike GT, Cravero JP, editors. *Pride, Prejudice and Pediatric Sedation: a multidisciplinary evaluation of the state of the art. Report from a Dartmouth Summit on Pediatric Sedation;* www.npsf.org/download/PediatricSedation.pdf (accessed 20 April 2007).

13 Advanced Life Support Group. *Advanced Paediatric Life Support: the practical approach.* 4th ed. London: BMJ Publishing; 2005.

14 Royal College of Anaesthetists, Association of Paediatric Anaesthetists and the Royal College of Paediatrics and Child Health. *Child Protection and the Anaesthetist: safeguarding children in the operating theatre (quick reference);* www.rcoa.ac.uk/apagbi/index.asp?SectionID=6 (accessed 17 June 2007).

15 HM Government. *Working Together to Safeguard Children;* www.everychildmatters.gov.uk/workingtogether (accessed 7 July 2007).

16 HM Government. *Children Act 1989;* www.opsi.gov.uk/acts/acts1989/Ukpga_19890041_en_1.htm (accessed 7 July 2007).

17 HM Government. *Children Act 2004;* www.opsi.gov.uk/acts/acts2004/20040031.htm (accessed 7 July 2007).

18 Sury MJ. Paediatric sedation. Continuing education in anaesthesia. *Crit Care Pain.* 2004; **4:** 118–22.

19 Litman RS, Kottra JA, Verga KA *et al.* Chloral hydrate sedation: the additive sedative and respiratory depressant effects of nitrous oxide. *Anesth Analg.* 1998; **86:** 724–8.

20 Louon A, Reddy VG. Nasal midazolam and ketamine for paediatric sedation during computerised tomography. *Acta Anaesthesiol Scand.* 1994; **38:** 259–61.

21 Cohen VG, Krauss B. Recurrent episodes of intractable laryngospasm during disassociative sedation with intramuscular ketamine. *Pediatr Emerg Care.* 2006; **22:** 247–9.

22 Mitchel RK, Koury SI, Stone CK. Respiratory arrest after intramuscular ketamine in a 2-year-old. *Am J Emerg Med.* 1996; **29:** 834–5.

23 Lawson GR, Bray RJ. Sedation of children for magnetic resonance imaging. *Arch Dis Child.* 2000; **82:** 150–4.

24 Davis C, Razavi R, Baker EJ. Sedation versus anaesthesia for MRI scanning in children. *Arch Dis Child.* 2000; **83:** 276–9.

25 Dearlove O, Corcoran JP. Sedation of children undergoing magnetic resonance imaging. *Br J Anaesth.* 2007; **98:** 548.

26 Sury MRJ, Hatch DJ, Millen W *et al.* The debate between sedation and anaesthesia for children undergoing MRI. *Arch Dis Child.* 2000; **83:** 276–9.

27 Royal Pharmaceutical Society of Great Britain. *The British National Formulary for Children.* London: BMJ Publishing; 2005.

CHAPTER 8

Sedation and the elderly

Increasing age is an independent risk factor for mortality and morbidity following medical interventions. However, chronological age alone is not the consistent, quantifiable risk factor that it may at first sight seem to be. Although subjectively we might agree that the older a patient is, the more at risk they are of complications or consequences of the effects of a medical procedure, it is not always possible to express this as a reliable odds ratio of harm. For example, everyone will be familiar with the 60-year-old person who 'looks older than their years' and who has limited activity compared with other people of the same age and, in contrast, the sprightly 90-year-old who still goes hill running. The athletic 90-year-old could be regarded as 'younger' than his nonagenarian counterparts, and the 60-year-old as 'older' than his cohort. This perception is often expressed in terms of *physiological age* as opposed to chronological age. This concept is useful when considering the risks of being elderly, in that it relates health to function and activity. However, at present the concept can only be used with regard to quantifying an individual's activity as better, the same as or worse than that which would normally be expected for someone of similar age. Investigators are currently evaluating more scientific ways of assessing this concept using objective tests such as the determination of *anaerobic exercise tolerance* levels. Current research in this area is extremely promising, as it appears that a low anaerobic threshold (AT) – that is, the activity level at which anaerobic metabolism starts – is associated with a quantifiably higher risk of mortality from major surgery. However, the technique is still in its infancy, and has not been applied to patients undergoing minor procedures.[1]

The physiology of ageing

After the age of 30 years, changes associated with ageing begin to develop, progressively affecting every organ and bodily system. The lungs become less elastic, and atelectasis can begin to occur even when the patient is sitting or standing, as the *closing volume* (the volume at which areas of collapse appear within the lungs) increases and encroaches upon normal functional lung volumes. This effect is exacerbated by general anaesthesia and lying down. Responses to hypoxia and hypercapnia are reduced, and protective airway reflexes are attenuated. Cardiac pacemaker activity and responsiveness decline, contributing to the generation of arrhythmias. Atrial fibrillation is particularly common in the elderly, and is regarded by some as a 'default rhythm' triggered by stress. Even without overt vascular disease, the vascular tree becomes 'stiffer', resulting in higher blood pressure and increased cardiac workload. This leads to left ventricular hypertrophy, predisposing to heart failure. Renal and liver function deteriorate. Cerebral blood flow is reduced, and parts of the brain are subject to atrophy. Confusion can become more common, particularly after surgical intervention. Muscle mass declines, and the metabolic rate generally decreases.

As a result, the elderly may respond differently to medication compared with their younger counterparts, because the way in which drugs are handled by the body can be altered. For example, age-related reductions in total body water mean that an equivalent dose of a water-soluble drug may be more concentrated within the tissues than expected. Alternatively, reduced drug metabolism may mean that exaggerated or prolonged action results.[2,3]

Assessing elderly patients

In addition to the normal process of ageing, physiology in the elderly may be affected by illness or concurrent medication. The pre-operative assessment of the elderly patient must therefore be aimed at identifying the presence of coexisting illness, as with any other patient, and also at determining their 'physiological age.' This can be assumed to be related to their *functionality*. The National Confidential Enquiry into Patient Outcome and Death (NCEPOD) found that 57% of elderly patients who had presented for surgery with an ultimately fatal outcome had a pre-existing cardiac pathology, and 28% had a respiratory disease.[4]

Specific scoring systems have been developed to assess risk in particular groups of patients, although their value in determining risk for an individual is disputed. Searching questions enquiring about normal activity levels may therefore be of more use in this context. For example, it is well known that patients with chronic illness may increasingly limit their activity in order to prevent symptoms. Enquiring about normal daily activities is a good way to determine this exercise tolerance. Asking patients how far they can walk on level ground without stopping, or whether they can walk around a supermarket without becoming short of breath are semi-quantitative in this respect. Patients may admit to being unable to walk down the garden path, or even around their bedroom, without symptoms. It must also be appreciated that disease in the elderly may present with a different spectrum of symptoms to those found in younger patients. For example, ischaemic heart disease may present with breathlessness rather than with angina.

Although one is unlikely to be able to declare that a patient's physiological age is, for example, '10 years younger' than their chronological one, an elderly patient who can climb a flight of stairs without stopping and without symptoms is likely to be at lower risk than one who cannot. It may be useful to watch an elderly person walk around the room in order to make a crude assessment of their exercise tolerance. If there is a suggestion of respiratory illness, a peak flow estimation can be performed. A normal peak flow is dependent upon good lung and respiratory muscle function. However, if peak flow data are not available, the ability (or inability) to count to 10 in one breath, or to blow out a match, can also provide useful information, as a patient who cannot perform these simple tests has poor lung function. If there is a suggestion of chronic lung disease, a pulse oximeter can be used to determine the patient's normal resting oxygen saturation.

TABLE 8.1 A typical cardiac risk score. Figures relate to risk of myocardial infarction or death during or after surgery

CONDITION	MAJOR RISK (> 5%)	INTERMEDIATE RISK (1–5%)	MINOR RISK (< 1%)
Ischaemic heart disease	MI < 1 month Unstable/severe angina	Previous MI Stable angina	Abnormal ECG
Congestive cardiac failure	Decompensated	Compensated (optimal treatment)	Reduced exercise capacity
Arrhythmia	Malignant SVT/VT Heart block		Abnormal (e.g. atrial fibrillation)
Other	Severe valvular disease	Diabetes	Uncontrolled hypertension

MI, myocardial infarction; ECG, electrocardiogram; SVT/VT, supraventricular tachycardia/ventricular tachycardia.

Cardiac symptoms can also be assessed and quantified using measures of exercise tolerance, or specific scoring systems, such as the Goldman score. Essentially this score, and those derived from it, assign a numerical value to the presence of various cardiac problems. The higher the score, the more at risk the patient may be of cardiac complications. A typical cardiac risk score is shown in Table 8.1.[5]

Cardiac risk scores are all essentially very similar. The presence of a recent heart attack, increasingly frequent angina, or heart failure are all indicators of high risk, and suggest that a cardiological review is necessary to ensure that symptoms are as stable as possible before the procedure takes place (*see* Box 8.1).

BOX 8.1 The importance of a stable cardiac rhythm

A surgeon asked an anaesthetist colleague whether it would be possible to administer an anaesthetic to an elderly patient who had 'reacted badly' when a gastroscopy had been attempted under sedation. During the sedation, he had 'dropped his saturations' and become breathless and tachycardic, but he recovered soon after the procedure was abandoned. Examination of the case notes revealed no abnormality except for a pre-procedure ECG, which demonstrated slow atrial fibrillation. It became obvious that the assumption had been made that the arrhythmia was a chronic condition, whereas in fact an ECG from the previous year had demonstrated a normal sinus rhythm. The patient had recent-onset atrial fibrillation that required investigation and stabilisation before the procedure could take place. An urgent cardiological review resulted in the control of the arrhythmia, and soon afterwards the patient successfully underwent an uneventful examination under sedation as originally planned.

The presence of a heart murmur may require a pre-sedation echocardiogram to exclude significant aortic stenosis, which can be associated with sudden collapse and death. The use of a pacemaker or an implantable cardiac defibrillator (ICD) will need specific consideration, as the function of these devices can be dramatically affected by intra-operative events, such as the use of diathermy. If presented with a patient who has such a device, the sedationist must determine the indication for its insertion, and when it was last checked, as it may be necessary for the pacemaker or ICD to be re-checked pre- and post-operatively by the local cardiac physiology department. Fortunately, such patients should always be carrying documentation in relation to this. The recent insertion of a coronary artery stent for ischaemic heart disease can make the patient a very high-risk candidate for any kind of intervention.

A good history with regard to the patient's daily activities can be extremely useful, as this can be expressed in terms of *metabolic equivalent levels (METs)*, as shown in Table 8.2. METs can be determined from treadmill tests, but have been validated in terms of everyday tasks.[6] One MET is the energy expenditure level required for the performance of basic functions, and the risk associated with surgery has been shown to decrease significantly if the patient can achieve a level of 4 METs or higher. However, it should be remembered that activity in the elderly can be reduced by factors which limit mobility, such as arthritis or claudication, as opposed to poor physiological reserve.

TABLE 8.2 Metabolic equivalent level of daily activities

METABOLIC LEVEL	EQUIVALENT ACTIVITY
1 MET	Eat
	Dress
	Use toilet
	Walk around house
	Do light housework
	Walk at a speed of 2–3 mph on level ground
4 METs	Climb one flight of ordinary stairs
	Walk uphill
	Run a short distance
	Do heavy housework
	Walk on level ground at a speed of 4 mph
	Recreational activity (golf, dancing, etc.)
6–7 METs	Short run
10 METs	Strenuous sports (swimming, skiing, football, etc.)

Once the assessment is complete, the sedationist should make a judgement of the suitability of the patient for the proposed procedure compared with the possible risks. Any suggestion of excess risk may warrant the presence of an anaesthetist during the procedure.

Specific advice with regard to sedation in the elderly

Sedation in the elderly has recently been the subject of two publications from national authorities in the UK. The National Confidential Enquiry into Patient Outcome and Death[7] (NCEPOD) considered the cases of over 1800 inpatients who had been subject to an endoscopic gastrointestinal investigational procedure within 30 days before death. In 14% of cases the assessors considered that the sedation method that had been used was incorrect, usually due to excessive drug dosages. This most often involved the administration of an inappropriately large dose of benzodiazepine, or a smaller dose being administered too quickly. The use of flumazenil to reverse the effects of benzodiazepine (an indication of inadvertent overdose) was associated with earlier death. Sadly, this finding was not new, as the association between dosage of benzodiazepine administered for sedation and death had been recognised nearly 10 years previously.[8] In addition, it was found that the monitoring used was deficient in 23% of cases considered, despite the fact that many of the patients who were undergoing procedures were unwell or undergoing emergency treatment.

It was also clear that because of altered physiological processes, the elderly are more vulnerable to the effects of sedative drugs (*see* Box 8.2). The National Patient Safety Agency (NPSA) therefore suggested that in patients over the age of 70 years, the expected maximum dose of midazolam calculated on a mg/kg basis should be halved, and given in increments until the desired effect is achieved, rather than as a single bolus dose. In fact, it was finally recommended that a maximum dose of 2 mg midazolam administered intravenously to patients over the age of 70 years would be sufficient in most cases, and it was stated specifically that in order to ensure this, no more than 2 mg should be drawn up into a syringe at any one time. The practice of drawing up the whole 10 mg of midazolam from the ampoule was condemned outright. In addition, if pethidine was to be used as part of the sedative technique, no more than 25 mg should be drawn up at any one time. Furthermore, it was suggested that manufacturers should explore the possibility of marketing ampoules that contain these specific dosages.[9]

BOX 8.2 Injudicious use of sedation in the elderly

The anaesthetic on-call team of a district general hospital was 'crash called' to the endoscopy suite. A woman in her seventies had been undergoing a colonoscopic procedure when it was realised that she had stopped breathing, and the endoscopy team had experienced difficulty in maintaining her airway. The anaesthetists controlled the patient's breathing and found that the woman, who weighed 65 kg, had been given 7 mg of midazolam by the sedationist as a single intravenous bolus because 'that is what I always do.' Administration of flumazenil resolved the situation, but the procedure was abandoned and the patient was admitted to the high-dependency unit for observation. The sedationist claimed to be unaware of the existing local guidelines about the use of intravenous sedation. The patient survived and underwent the procedure again at a later date, when midazolam was given in a smaller dose, titrated to effect.

Resuscitation

Resuscitation of the elderly should adhere to the same guidelines and standards as for any other adult. However, the outcome of cardiac arrest in the elderly is poor, and patients over the age of 80 years tend not to survive prolonged ITU stays.

Summary

The sedation of elderly patients requires consideration of the added risks that are associated with age and coexisting illness. The sedationist should be aware that the elderly will often require a reduced dosage of sedation, and he or she will need to be alert to the possibility of complications which can arise from chronic illness or related treatments.

LEARNING POINTS

- Sedation in the elderly involves additional hazards compared with sedation in younger adults.
- A good history of the patient's functionality is required in order to make an accurate assessment of risk.
- A reduced dosage of sedative drugs is recommended.

References

1 Older P, Hall A, Hader R. Cardiopulmonary exercise testing as a screening test for perioperative management of major surgery in the elderly. *Chest.* 1999; **116:** 355–62.

2 Vaughn S. The elderly patient. In: McConachie I, editor. *Anaesthesia for the High-Risk Patient.* London: Greenwich Medical Media; 2002.

3 Association of Anaesthetists of Great Britain and Ireland. *Anaesthesia and*

Peri-Operative Care of the Elderly. London: Association of Anaesthetists of Great Britain and Ireland; 2001.

4 National Confidential Enquiry into Patient Outcome and Death. *Extremes of Age. The 1999 Report of the National Confidential Enquiry into Peri-Operative Death*; www. ncepod.org.uk/1999.htm (accessed 9 August 2007).

5 Day C. Cardiovascular disease. In: Allman KG, Wilson IH, editors. *The Oxford Handbook of Anaesthesia.* Oxford: Oxford University Press; 2001.

6 Hlatky MA. Boineau RE, Higginbotham MB *et al.* A brief self-administered questionnaire to determine functional capacity (the Duke Activity Status Index). *Am J Cardiol.* 1989: **64:** 651–4.

7 National Confidential Enquiry into Patient Outcome and Death. *Scoping Our Practice*; www.ncepod.org.uk/pdf/2004/04sum.pdf (accessed 11 February 2007).

8 Quine MA, Bell GD, McCloy RF *et al.* Prospective audit of upper gastrointestinal endoscopy in two regions of England: safety, staffing and sedation methods. *Gut.* 1995; **36:** 462–7.

9 Gray A, Bell GD. *Elderly Patients Vulnerable Because of Excessive Doses of Sedatives*; www.ncepod.org.uk/pdf/current/NPSA sedation article.pdf (accessed 31 March 2007).

CHAPTER 9

Sedation in community dental practice

The history of modern anaesthesia is entwined with the history of modern dental practice, and it is therefore fitting that it is developments in dental sedation and anaesthesia that have led the way in setting standards for sedation across the healthcare sector. A brief summary of the history of dental anaesthetic practice is therefore relevant.

A brief history of dental anaesthetic practice

Modern anaesthesia started with the search for a painless method of enabling dental extraction. Horace Wells, an American dentist, utilised nitrous oxide (N_2O) for this purpose from 1844. Soon other agents, such as the volatile liquids chloroform and ether, were also utilised. The success of these gases in dentistry stimulated interest in their use for other types of surgery.

Although the administration of anaesthetics within hospital practice in the UK tended to be performed only by physicians, in community dental practice the situation was different. 'Dental-chair' anaesthesia continued to a large extent to be given by experienced dental surgeons as well as by doctors. In some cases the anaesthetist and the operator were the same person.

In the late 1980s and early 1990s, several cases of unexpected deaths during dental treatment led to a public outcry. These fatalities were particularly tragic as the patients were generally previously fit and well children undergoing simple elective treatment. The deaths were often associated with poorly thought out procedures, performed by poorly trained individuals working in environments that were not fit for purpose, using anaesthesia as a means of reducing anxiety. In other words, the fatalities were totally preventable.[1,2]

Investigation showed that certain anaesthetic agents predisposed to cardiac arrhythmia, and the hazards of cardiovascular collapse were exacerbated by the upright positioning of the child in the dental chair. Furthermore, vasovagal attacks and arrhythmias were associated with stimulation of the trigeminal nerve by the surgeon.[3–5] The so-called Poswillo Report[6] recommended major changes in dental anaesthetic practice across the UK, leading to more procedures being performed in a hospital environment. The recommendations of the report are summarised in Table 9.1. By 2002, the provision of anaesthesia in community dental practices was effectively banned.[7,8] However, it was recognised that there was a huge demand for some method of facilitating dental treatment in the community setting which effectively alleviated anxiety. If all patients who were fearful about dental treatment were referred to hospitals for anaesthetics, the infrastructure would not be able to cope with the demand.

TABLE 9.1 The Poswillo Report recommendations with regard to anaesthetic practice in dental surgeries

Anaesthesia

Anaesthesia in dental surgeries is a postgraduate subject.

The use of general anaesthesia should be avoided wherever possible. All anaesthetics should be administered or at least supervised by an accredited anaesthetist.

The appropriate standards of personnel, premises, monitoring and equipment required apply wherever general anaesthesia is administered. A defibrillator must be available.

Intravenous agents should be administered via an indwelling cannula or needle, which is to remain *in situ* until the patient is fully awake.

There should be adequate facilities for recovery, and the recovering patient should not be left unattended.

All patients should receive written post-procedure instructions, and be escorted home by a responsible adult.

All staff should be trained in resuscitation.

Sedation

Sedation should be used in preference to general anaesthesia.

For sedation, the *minimum* administered oxygen concentration is 30%.

Flumazenil is reserved for emergency usage, and is not a standard part of a sedative technique.

Intravenous sedation should be limited to one drug titrated to an end point remote from anaesthesia. Intravenous sedation should be used with caution in children.

More emphasis should be given to training in sedation.

The Poswillo recommendations have since been further refined by a variety of bodies (*see* Table 9.2).

TABLE 9.2 Summary of the recommendations of the Expert Group on Sedation for Dentistry, 2003[9]

The effective management of pain and anxiety is of paramount importance for patients undergoing dentistry. *Conscious sedation is an essential component of this and, when competently provided, it is safe, valuable and effective.*

A wide margin of safety must be maintained between conscious sedation and the unconscious state of general anaesthesia. *Conscious sedation must not under any circumstances be interpreted as light general anaesthesia.*

A high level of competence is required, based upon a solid foundation of theoretical and practical supervised training, progressive updating of skills, and continuing practice. *This applies to* all *members of the dental team, and includes training in the management of complications.*

Various societies for the promotion of safe practice in dental anaesthesia have existed for some time, e.g. the Society for the Advancement of Anaesthesia in Dentistry (www.saaduk.org). These organisations have worked hard to maintain the practice of sedation as an identifiable and separate entity in the primary care dental setting. The Dental Sedation Teachers Group (www. dstg.co.uk) has been working to establish UK-wide standards for training in dental sedation.

Safe practice of dental sedation in the community

The principles of safe practice for dental sedation are the same as those for sedation in any other environment, but the available emergency facilities may be very different from those in a hospital setting. For example, a so-called 'crash team' is not available if assistance is required in an unexpected emergency. It is the understanding of these differences that defines the competencies which are essential for a sedationist working outside the hospital environment.

Standards of sedation in dentistry

The definition of sedation given by the General Dental Council (GDC) is the same as that previously defined in Chapter 1. The standards for practice are reiterated in many GDC documents,[10,11] and are summarised in Table 9.3. These and other documents specifically recommend that general anaesthesia, including deep sedation, should not be practised outside the hospital environment.[12–14]

TABLE 9.3 Professional standards for anaesthesia in dental practice

Dental treatment under anaesthesia should only take place when it is judged to be the most appropriate method. It should only occur in a hospital setting with critical care facilities available.

General anaesthesia should only be given by someone who is on the GMC specialist register as an anaesthetist, or who is a trainee working under supervision on a Royal College of Anaesthetists-approved training programme, or who is a non-consultant career grade doctor working under the auspices of a named consultant anaesthetist employed at the same department.

The anaesthetist should be supported by someone who is specifically trained and experienced in the skills necessary to help to monitor the patient's condition and assist in any emergency.

It should be noted that the GDC places specific duties on the treating *dentist* to ensure that the sedationist is properly trained and using appropriate techniques, and to ensure that the dental team are fully conversant with emergency treatment measures. This is illustrated by the case in Box 9.1.

BOX 9.1 The dentist's responsibilities

Patient A, a 6-year-old boy, attended a dental surgery to have multiple extractions. The sedation was given by an anaesthetist who administered a cocktail of drugs in bolus fashion, rather than titrating to effect. The child became cyanosed in the recovery area and, despite emergency treatment, was left with brain damage. An inquiry revealed that essential equipment was not available, and that staff were unfamiliar with emergency guidelines. The dentist was struck off the register for, among other things, failing to 'rehearse emergency procedures, including life support techniques with the members of the dental team' and failing to 'ensure that the sedationist accepted the principle of minimum intervention.'

Dentist fights for job after drugs blunder; www.cambridge-news.co.uk/news/city/2006/10/05/de7944b7-f263-46ff-926e-aa38f2cd8f67.lpf (accessed 13 June 2007).

www.gdc-uk.org/GDC/Templates?Forms?Hearingsummary.aspx (accessed 13 June 2007).

The purpose of sedation in dentistry is threefold:

1 to reduce anxiety and maintain the patient's comfort and cooperation
2 to facilitate treatment
3 to prevent the creation/exacerbation of a 'dental phobia.'

Dental phobia

This is the term used to describe excessive fear of undergoing dental treatment. It is an anxiety common to many people, but can be a debilitating problem in a large number of patients. Not only can such a fear prevent patients from accessing dental treatment, but it can also have significant effects on other aspects of their lives.[15] Despite this, when questioned about preferences, 65% of patients would prefer to be conscious if they could be pain-free during dental treatment, with 56% of respondents also wishing for amnesia.[16] Much can be done to alleviate the feelings of anxiety, and a well-planned intervention, explained and performed by professional staff in a friendly environment, may well obviate the requirement for sedation altogether. Exploring the exact nature of the fear may make it possible for the patient to undergo a dental procedure without sedation. For example, if the patient fears the sight of the drill, reassurance and dark glasses may be sufficient to allow procedures to occur. Behavioural therapy, hypnosis and acupuncture have all been recorded as helping to avoid the need for pharmacological sedation. Sedation, like any other medical intervention, should only be utilised when necessary.

Much work has been done to try to create a validated anxiety scoring scale which can be used to aid research in this area.[17]

The operator-sedationist

In some circumstances, the individual who is administering the sedation and the surgeon who is performing the dental work may be one and the same person, in which case they are referred to as the 'operator-sedationist.' A practitioner who assumes this dual role must ensure that the monitoring of the patient is delegated to a suitably trained person who can assist in the event of a complication.[14]

Training and skills in dental sedation

It is assumed that the new sedationist will initially be working under supervision in an appropriate environment, and will keep and maintain a logbook as proof of training and experience.[18] The full knowledge base and skills needed are dealt with in detail in other chapters. However, the sedationist must be able to assess patients appropriately, ensure that the environment is safe, obtain consent, choose an appropriate sedation technique, be technically proficient, and ensure that the patient has recovered fully. A case mix of 100 patients per annum has been suggested as a reasonable number to keep skills current.[19]

The sedationist skills required can vary according to the sedation technique employed – that is, whether the route of administration is *inhalational*, *intravenous* or *oral*. Much research is being done into the efficacy of oral sedation in community paediatric dental practice. However, a dose of 0.3 mg/kg midazolam has been compared favourably with nitrous oxide inhalation.[20] Oral sedation can be very effective, but may require a considerable amount of time to take effect.

Inhalational sedation should only be administered to patients from a purpose-designed relative analgesia machine that meets appropriate British Standards.[21] Although sedation using volatile anaesthetic agents in combination with intravenous sedation and nitrous oxide has been proposed,[22] the use of such techniques should be confined to hospital practice by trained anaesthetists. Nitrous oxide in oxygen is the only universally approved inhalational dental sedation technique for children under 16 years of age. One method of using nitrous oxide is to administer pure oxygen to the patient for up to 5 minutes, and then slowly introduce the nitrous oxide until the desired effect is reached. Dental surgeries that utilise inhalational sedation must conform to appropriate standards, as chronic exposure to nitrous oxide can have health implications for staff.[23]

Intravenous sedation should normally be confined to the use of one drug, usually midazolam, titrated to effect rather than administered as a bolus. Intravenous sedation is not recommended for children under the age of 16 years. However, although intravenous midazolam has been utilised in conjunction with inhalational techniques, it should be remembered that much of this research originates from outside the UK, and therefore may not be directly applicable to UK practice. Newer drugs such as dexmedetomidine have been used for this purpose in the USA, where that particular drug is reported to maintain respiratory parameters, although low blood pressure and slow heart rate may result.[17] Increasing research in this context is also being conducted with propofol.

The sedationist has a duty to use a technique that is suitable for the patient, but also has a duty to adhere to acceptable standards of practice, taking reasonable steps to avoid the inadvertent induction of anaesthesia (*see* Box 9.2). However, despite prolific research in this field, it is not yet possible to recommend the use of one technique over another on an evidential basis.[24] Guidelines therefore usually recommend what is *believed* to be safe.

> **BOX 9.2 Consequences of poor dental sedation techniques**
>
> A dental clinic was subject to several complaints with regard to the sedation services supplied by Dr B. It was alleged that a variety of incidents occurred, which included a young girl being left on a fire escape to recover from her sedation, and a young boy allegedly suffering brain damage. At a GMC hearing, his sedation technique, which involved a combination of ketamine, alfentanil and midazolam, was described as 'an accident waiting to happen.'
>
> GMC hears drugged children charge; http://news.bbc.co.uk/1/hi/england/cambridgeshire/4852734.stm (accessed 25 April 2006).
>
> Boy vomited blood after dental surgery; www.cambridge-news.co.uk/news/city (accessed 25 April 2006).
>
> Boy 'brain damaged in dental sedation'; www.cambridge-news.co.uk/news/city (accessed 25 April 2006).

Hazards of dental sedation

Sedation for dental practice has some features which may not be shared with other clinical specialties. For example, the patient mix can be very eclectic. A large proportion of the patients are children, and are fit and well. Another significant proportion may have physical or mental impairment which prevents them from cooperating readily with dental treatment, while others will be adults with severe anxiety issues. All of these patients will have specific needs which the dental team will need to address.

Patients may be sedated in an upright sitting position in the dental chair, which means that an unexpected drop in blood pressure from whatever cause can lead to excessive difficulties. For this reason, the sedationist should be sure that the chair can be moved to a horizontal position in a crisis. In addition, the patient's airway is shared between the surgeon and the sedationist, which may lead to difficulty in managing respiration if the patient becomes deeply sedated, particularly if there is heavy soiling of the oral cavity by the dentist.

It has been suggested that in some cases, such as pure inhalational sedation, the need for the patient to be fasted and the requirement for full monitoring may not be necessary.[25] However, one of the recurrent problems with 'dental-chair' anaesthetic deaths was that practitioners 'had an almost magical belief that somehow this type of anaesthesia was different to that in a hospital, and was without harm',[2] so such recommendations should be treated with the utmost caution. It is worth remembering that there is no objective evidence to show that sedation is intrinsically safer than anaesthesia, but there is evidence that the presence of professional, appropriately trained staff in a properly equipped environment does make the difference between safe and unsafe sedation. Patients should be closely monitored at all times, and should be allowed to recover from sedation in an appropriately monitored area. The criteria for discharge are the same as those for any other day-case surgery patient. Patients, or their carers, should be given ample written information with regard to what action to take and who to contact if problems arise later on (*see* Box 9.3).

BOX 9.3 Inadequate sedation practice

A, a 4-year-old boy, underwent sedation at a dental practice under the care of Dr T. Dr T did not perform a proper pre-sedation assessment and failed either to detect or to record A's pre-existing illnesses. Initially nitrous oxide sedation was commenced, but this was inadequate, and midazolam was given. Dr T did not adequately record this, or the dosage administered. Dr T allowed A to be discharged from the clinic before he had fully recovered from the sedation. The parents were so concerned about A's condition that they took him straight to hospital. Dr T had conditions placed upon his registration by the General Medical Council.

de Sousa L. Boy given cocktail of drugs for dental treatment (21 December 2006); http://icberkshire.icnetwork.co.uk/0100news/0200berkshirehead lines/tm_headline=boy-given--cocktail-of-drugs-for-dental-treatment&m ethod=full&objectid=18309871&siteid=50102-name_page.html (accessed 15 August 2007).

de Sousa L. Doctor's apology for sending home unconscious 4-year-old boy (12 January 2007); http://icberkshire.icnetwork.co.uk/0100news/02 00berkshireheadlines/tm_headline=doctor-s-apology-for-sending-home-unconscious-four-year-old&method=full&objectid=18449961&siteid=5010 2-name_page.html (accessed 15 August 2007).

Summary

The standards that apply to sedation for dental practice have developed from well-documented disasters in dental-chair anaesthetic practice. Community dental practice has many risks which are unique to that environment, although it appears that the potential dangers may still be underestimated by some. Much work has been done to attempt to determine the nature of the appropriate skills and experience required to provide safe sedation for this work.

LEARNING POINTS

- The community dental practice environment has unique risks.
- The dentist is responsible for ensuring that the sedationist is appropriately trained and using appropriate techniques, and that the dental team is trained in appropriate resuscitation measures.
- The sedationist must ensure that they are appropriately trained, and that they are practising in an appropriate environment.

References

1 Cantlay K, Williamson S, Hawkings J. Anaesthesia for dentistry. *Contin Educ Anaesth. Crit Care Pain.* 2005; **5:** 71–5.

2 Strunin L. Intravenous conscious sedation for dental treatment: am I my brother's keeper? *Anaesthesia.* 2007; **62:** 645–7.

3 Worthington LM, Flynn PJ, Strunin L. Death in the dental chair: an avoidable catastrophe? *Anaesthesia.* 1998; **80:** 131–2.

4 Coplans MP, Curson I. Deaths associated with dentistry. *Br Dent J.* 1982; **153:** 357–62.

5 Coplans MP, Curson I. Deaths associated with dentistry and dental disease, 1980–1989. *Anaesthesia.* 1993; **48:** 435–8.

6 Poswillo D. *General Anaesthesia, Sedation and Resuscitation in Dentistry. Report of an Expert Working Party for the Standing Dental Advisory Committee.* London: Department of Health; 1990.

7 Lahoud GY. Death in the dental chair. *Anaesthesia.* 2000; **55:** 88–9.

8 Landes DP. The provision of general anaesthesia in dental practice: an end which had to come? *Br Dent J.* 2002; **192:** 129–31.

9 Standing Dental Advisory Committee. *Conscious Sedation in the Provision of Dental Care. Report of the Expert Group on Sedation for Dentistry;* www.doh.gov.uk/sdac (accessed 25 May 2007).

10 General Dental Council. *Maintaining Standards. Guidance to dentists, dental hygienists and dental therapists on professional and personal conduct.* London: General Dental Council; 1998 (amended 2001).

11 General Dental Council. *Standards for Dental Professionals*. London: General Dental Council; 2005.

12 Dental Sedation Teachers Group. *Training for Safe Practice in Advanced Sedation Techniques for Adult Patients*; www.dstg.co.uk/teaching/advanced-sedation (accessed 24 April 2007).

13 European Academy of Paediatric Dentistry. Curriculum guidelines for education and training in paediatric dentistry. *Int J Paediatr Dent.* 1997; **7**: 273–81.

14 Scottish Dental Clinical Effectiveness Programme. *Conscious Sedation in Dentistry. Dental clinical guidance*; www.scottishdental.org/cep/docs/Concious_Sedation_in_Dentistry.pdf (accessed 24 June 2007).

15 Cohen SM, Fiske J, Newton JT. The impact of dental anxiety on daily living. *Br Dent J.* 2000; **189**: 385–90.

16 Delfino J. Public attitudes toward oral surgery: results of a Gallup poll. *J Oral Maxillofac Surg.* 1997; **55**: 564–7.

17 Leitch J, Macpherson A. Current state of sedation/analgesia care in dentistry. *Curr Opin Anaesthesiol.* 2007; **20**: 384–7.

18 Dental Sedation Teachers Group. *Sedation in Dentistry: the competent graduate*; www.dstg.co.uk/teaching/competent-graduate/ (accessed 2 August 2007).

19 Dental Sedation Teachers Group. *Training in Conscious Sedation in Dentistry*; www.dstg.co.uk/teaching/tics-2005/DSTG%20TICS%202005.doc (accessed 12 June 2007).

20 Wilson KE, Girdler NM, Welbury RR. A comparison of oral midazolam and nitrous oxide sedation for dental extractions in children. *Anaesthesia.* 2006; **61**: 1138–44.

21 British Standards Institute. *Anaesthetic and Analgesic Machines. BS4273.* London: British Standards Institute; 1997.

22 Averley PA, Girdler NM, Bond S *et al.* A randomised controlled trial of paediatric conscious sedation for dental treatment using intravenous midazolam combined with inhaled nitrous oxide/sevoflurane. *Anaesthesia.* 2004; **59**: 844–52.

23 Health Expert Advisory Committee. *Anaesthetic Agents: controlling exposure under COSHH.* London: Health Expert Advisory Committee; 1995.

24 Matharu L, Ashley PF. *Sedation of Anxious Children Undergoing Dental Treatment. Cochrane Review Database*; www.cochrane.org/reviews/en/ab003877.html (accessed 3 August 2007).

25 Hallonsten A-L, Jensen B, Raadal JM *et al. EAPD Guideline on Sedation in Paediatric Dentistry*; www.eapd.gr/Guidelines/EAPD_sedation_guidelines-_final.pdf (accessed 13 June 2007).

CHAPTER 10

Sedation for radiological procedures

Many procedures that were previously only possible with surgery and a full anaesthetic are now feasible utilising minimally invasive procedures under radiological control. These procedures usually take place in dedicated suites, sometimes quite distant from anaesthetic and other support. A selection of these procedures is listed in Table 10.1.

TABLE 10.1 Procedures commonly performed under radiological control

- Cardiovascular procedures:
  - Balloon angioplasty
  - Stenting of diseased vessels
  - Thrombectomy
  - Thrombolysis
  - Embolisation
- Central line placement
- Renal vascular access procedures
- Neuroradiology:
  - Coiling of cerebral aneurysms

Although the field of interventional radiology is rapidly expanding, the specialties of interventional cardiology and neuroradiology are also developing a growing patient base, and usually require the rapid throughput of high-risk patients.

All of these procedures carry their own risks, irrespective of any complications which may arise from sedation. However, there is a common hazard to staff and patients from exposure to radiation and magnetic fields. Sedationists have a key role in ensuring that they and their patients are protected from unnecessary exposure. This will include determining whether female patients could be pregnant and, if they are, taking appropriate precautions (e.g. warning radiology staff; covering the abdomen with a lead jacket, etc.). There is also a probability that in some circumstances the sedationist may have to remain isolated from the patient.

Radiation protection

The use of radiation is governed by very strict regulations[1] under which the employer is responsible for protecting staff, patients and the public, and for monitoring and maintaining equipment. The intensity of exposure is subject to the inverse square rule – that is, the amount of radiation present is inversely proportional to the square of the distance that one is from the source. In other words, the further away one is from the source, the less radiation there is. Therefore the simplest protective measure that staff can use is distance. Lead shielding is available to improve personal protection and, failing this, staff should stand behind appropriate fixed or mobile shields. The patient can be protected by minimising exposure in relation to the extent of the body imaged, the intensity of radiation used, and the duration of exposure.

Standards for sedation practice in radiology departments were first formulated in 1992,[2] and have subsequently been revised as practice has changed in various subspecialties.[3]

The basic principles highlighted in these reports are shown in Table 10.2.

TABLE 10.2 Recommendations with regard to sedation in radiology departments

Sedation should be performed under the responsibility of a named consultant radiologist.
The person who is performing the intervention or imaging should not be the same individual who is responsible for administering and monitoring the sedation.
Responsibility for sedation should not be delegated to the trainee who is learning the radiological procedure, or the scrub nurse.
Anaesthetic assistance should be readily available when required.
Failed sedation should not be converted to anaesthesia on the same day. The procedure should be abandoned, and the patient should be listed for an anaesthetic.
A radiology department in which sedation is performed should be equipped to the same standard as those areas in the hospital where anaesthesia is performed.
All staff should be trained in and maintain their competency in resuscitation techniques.

Specific issues

Simple imaging

It is unlikely that many patients will require sedation for simple radiographic imaging. Trauma patients or those from ITU will be either anaesthetised, or at least accompanied by an anaesthetist if they are thought to be at risk. Patients who are undergoing painful procedures (e.g. the insertion of chest drains, or the drainage of abscesses under ultrasound control) may be managed with reassurance and local anaesthesia in most cases. Patients who are undergoing the biopsy of a solid organ (e.g. a kidney) may require anaesthesia if they are uncooperative.

CT scanning

Computerised tomography (CT) scanning involves the patient being placed inside a large ring which subjects the body to X-rays from several directions at once. The sedationist can remain in the scanner room with the patient if he or she is appropriately shielded. Modern CT scanners can complete a study within a few minutes. If sedation is performed, care must be taken that monitoring leads or equipment do not interfere with the image, and do not become damaged when the table or the ring move in relation to each other.

MRI scanning[4]

Magnetic resonance imaging (MRI) involves the use of a strong magnetic field of the order of 0.3 tesla or above to change the spinning properties of hydrogen atoms. The resulting change of atom phases is analysed in order to obtain detailed images. These devices are large, and involve sliding the patient completely inside a cylinder. Due to the powerful effects of the magnetic field on ferromagnetic substances, the MRI scanners often have to be housed inside specially designed buildings in order to protect the staff and the public. The full effects of powerful magnetic fields on the human body have not yet been fully evaluated.

Due to the startling detail of the images produced, the uses of the device have expanded. Some of the scanning processes, such as imaging of the spine, can take a considerable amount of time to complete.

There are several key issues to consider in this environment.

➠ The patient is isolated within the cylinder, and access is limited, which reduces the ability to return to the patient in a timely manner should a difficulty arise. In addition, the feeling of isolation experienced by the patient can induce anxiety and distress due to claustrophobia. There is some evidence that the magnetic field may affect the semicircular canals (causing vertigo and nausea) or the retina (causing 'flashing lights' to be seen). In addition, the noise produced by the scanner can cause real discomfort. Staff are usually housed within a special booth, remote from the patient, but the booth should have easy egress to the scanning area in case of emergency.

➡ The strength of the magnet is such that any ferromagnetic substance can be attracted to it with projectile force. This can include monitoring apparatus, anaesthetic equipment, trolleys and even oxygen cylinders. Therefore when a facility is being planned, account has to be taken of the fact that specialist equipment that is MRI compatible will need to be purchased in order to facilitate the management of anaesthetised and sedated patients. If this equipment is not available, it will not be possible to anaesthetise or sedate the patient in the MRI suite. It may not be possible for a sedationist to remain in the scanner area, so the facility to monitor the patient remotely should be available. In the case of ITU patients, this means that extra long intravenous lines and ventilator breathing circuits must be available.

➡ All personnel and patients who are being placed near the scanner need to be screened to ensure that they do not have any implanted ferromagnetic prostheses or devices. A pacemaker is a definite contraindication to undergoing such a scan.

➡ 'Quenching' of superconducting magnets is a rare but real danger. Quenching occurs when the MRI magnet is shut down. This may produce a risk of asphyxiation if the ventilation of the scanner room is inadequate, as rapid evaporation of the liquid helium used to cool the magnet may occur, and the vapour may escape. The scanner room should therefore be fitted with sensors which can provide early warning of this problem. The sedationist should be aware of the procedures that need to be followed in the event of such an emergency.

It can therefore be seen that the sedation technique employed for patients undergoing MRI scanning has to satisfy a variety of different criteria. Some authorities believe that this is one scenario in which anaesthesia is definitely safer than sedation.[5,6] However, some departments have successfully developed MRI sedation services involving non-anaesthetists. The most successful of these have been developed with the active cooperation of the anaesthetic department.[7]

General risks of interventional procedures

Interventional cardiological and neuroradiological procedures usually initially involve the cannulation of a major blood vessel under imaging control. The techniques that are utilised vary, but often involve a technique akin to that known as the 'Seldinger technique', in which a vessel is cannulated and then a guide wire is inserted. The guide wire is used to allow dilation of the vessel, followed by insertion of various catheters. The catheters can be used to allow the passage of instruments to perform a variety of procedures, once the vascular tree has been mapped using radio-opaque dye. As such, the main complications are always patient discomfort and the risk of bleeding from the punctured blood vessel, as well as damage to related structures. The use of radiological contrast media can precipitate a life-threatening allergic reaction. In addition, there is the possibility that any chronic condition affecting a patient (e.g. epilepsy) may deteriorate and cause a hazard during a procedure.

Neuroradiology

In neuroradiology, such techniques are often utilised to facilitate the treatment of vascular aneurysms by the insertion of a 'coil' which obliterates the abnormality. The main hazard is that the procedure could precipitate a catastrophic brain haemorrhage or a stroke.

Interventional cardiology

In recent years the specialty of cardiology has become increasingly interventional, with many procedures previously performed by cardiothoracic surgeons under anaesthesia now being performed under sedation in a *cardiac catheterisation laboratory (CCL)*. Some of the issues relating to these procedures, such as radiation hazards, have already been discussed in previous sections. However, there are a variety of procedures in this expanding and challenging field which need further consideration.

Patients who present as emergencies to CCLs for percutaneous coronary intervention (PCI) may well be haemodynamically unstable, and time constraints may dictate that there is little scope for improving the situation, as any increased delay to intervention results in the death of more cardiac muscle, and therefore a worsening of the situation. This risk may be increased when percutaneous valve correction is performed. It may well be that general anaesthesia is the best option in some circumstances. Even if the patient is stable, the possibility of a prolonged procedure, or other patient-related factors, may mean that anaesthesia should be considered. The possibility of a cardiac complication (e.g. an arrhythmia) occurring is quite high.

Electrophysiological procedures such as ablation may also be quite lengthy, as the mapping of aberrant conducting pathways may take several hours. The insertion of implantable defibrillators will require testing of the device *in situ*, which can be quite painful for the patient. Other interventions include the occlusion of septal defects, implantation of pacemakers, insertion of counter-pulsation balloon pumps and the use of invasive investigations such as transoesophageal echocardiology.

It has been acknowledged that the establishment of sedation procedures within a CCL requires close collaboration with the anaesthetic department, if only to ensure that there are clear lines of communication for quick access to anaesthetic opinion and assistance in an emergency.[8] Cardiac procedures of this type are also being performed increasingly on children under sedation. However, it should be remembered that much of the work in this field comes from North America, and refers to 'deep sedation' of children, a level of sedation that is defined as anaesthesia in the UK.[9]

Summary

Expansion of medical knowledge means that new techniques are being used to treat illnesses that were formerly traditionally cured by means of surgery and anaesthesia. Often these new approaches involve the use of radiological imaging techniques in isolated areas. Sedationists who are involved in such treatments should be part of a well-developed team, working to set guidelines.

LEARNING POINTS

- Many interventional and imaging procedures may require the use of sedation.
- The sedationist has an active role to play in the protection of staff and patients from radiation and other hazards.
- The standards that apply to sedation practice in such areas are the same as those that have been previously defined in Chapters 4 and 6.
- Sedation for MRI scanning will require specialist equipment.
- Individual interventional procedures can be associated with specific hazards.

References

1 Department of Health. *The Ionising Radiation (Medical Exposure) Regulations*; www.dh.gov.uk/prod_consum_dh/groups/dh_digitalassets/@dh/@en/ documents/digitalasset/dh_4057838.pdf (accessed 13 June 2007).

2 Royal College of Anaesthetists. *Sedation and Anaesthesia in Radiology. Recommendations of the Joint Working Party of the Royal College of Radiologists and the Royal College of Anaesthetists.* London: Royal College of Anaesthetists; 1992.

3 British Society of Neuroradiologists. *Effective Neuroradiology Guidelines for Safe and Efficient Practice*; www.bsnr.co.uk/Effective%20Neuroradiology.pdf (accessed 15 March 2007).

4 Association of Anaesthetists of Great Britain and Ireland. *Provision of Anaesthetic Services in Magnetic Resonance Units*; www.aagbi.org/publications/guidelines/ docs/mri02.pdf (accessed 25 May 2007).

5 Sury MRJ, Hatch DJ, Millen W *et al.* The debate between sedation and anaesthesia for children undergoing MRI. *Arch Dis Child.* 2000; **83**: 276–9.

6 Lawson GR, Bray RJ. Sedation of children for magnetic resonance imaging. *Arch Dis Child.* 2000; **82**: 150–4.

7 Dearlove O, Corcoran JP. Sedation of children undergoing magnetic resonance imaging. *Br J Anaesth.* 2007; **98**: 548 (letter).

8 Shook DC, Gross W. Offsite anaesthesiology in the cardiac catheterisation lab. *Curr Opin Anaesthesiol.* 2007; **20**: 352–8.

9 Hertzog JH, Havidich JE. Non-anaesthesiologist-provided pediatric procedural sedation: an update. *Curr Opin Anaesthesiol.* 2007; **20**: 365–72.

CHAPTER 11

Sedation in critical care

The Intensive-Care Unit (ICU) is a facility within which seriously unwell patients are treated with invasive supportive therapies, such as ventilation, inotropic support and dialysis. In 2000, the UK Government redefined such areas and affiliated wards (such as High-Dependency Units) as *Critical Care Units*.[1] That paper defined *critical care medicine* as a separate medical entity, and outlined the resources that need to be available to ensure that patients receive appropriate care in an appropriate environment. The paper defined these requirements as different 'levels of care.' These levels are described in Table 11.1.

TABLE 11.1 Definitions of different 'levels of care'

LEVEL	DESCRIPTION	EXAMPLE
0	Patients whose needs can be met through normal ward care in an acute hospital.	Inpatient under going day-case investigation, treatment, or minor to moderate surgery.
1	Patients at risk of their condition deteriorating, or those recently relocated from higher levels of care, whose needs can be met on an acute ward with additional advice and support from the critical care team.	Patients with serious underlying disease, or those who have had moderate to major surgery.
2	Patients who require more detailed observation or intervention, including support for a single failing organ system or post-operative care, and those 'stepping down' from higher levels of care.	Patients with single-organ failure (e.g. kidney failure).

cont.

LEVEL	DESCRIPTION	EXAMPLE
3	Patients who require advanced respiratory support alone, or basic respiratory support together with support of at least two organ systems. This level includes all complex patients who require support for multi-organ failure.	Traditional ICU patients on ventilators, or patients with more than single-organ failure.

Examination of these definitions shows that specialist areas within a hospital, such as medical admission units, theatre recovery areas, renal units, and so on, can be classified using this scale. For the purposes of this discussion, we shall assume that we are referring only to 'Level 3' patients who require ventilatory support, or who have single- or multiple-organ failure, on an ICU.

Analgesia and sedation on the ICU

The purpose of the ICU is to support the physiological function of those patients with serious illness who are thought to have a good chance of recovery. These patients often require invasive, painful or distressing treatment for days, and so need to be able to tolerate these therapies. Therefore sedation is often required to maintain the patient's comfort. However, sedation in the ICU is a specialist skill, as the patients often have disordered physiology, and therefore unpredictable pharmacological responses. For example, the serum albumin level is often low, which may alter the active proportion of a drug that is available, and thereby alter the drug's effect.

Analgesia

Analgesia for ICU patients must be considered separately to their sedation needs. Some patients will require pain relief because they have undergone surgery, or are victims of trauma. However, others may require some analgesia in order to tolerate an indwelling endotracheal tube, or the discomfort of positive pressure ventilation. Although some analgesics will have sedative side-effects, they should *in most circumstances be prescribed only for analgesic purposes*.

Analgesia can be achieved using local anaesthetic or systemic opiates. Local anaesthetic is an excellent way of achieving post-operative pain relief, and can be given either as a 'one-off' shot after operation, as an infusion through an indwelling cannula (for a specific continuous nerve block), or through an epidural catheter. Many epidural medication mixtures now contain a combination of low-concentration local anaesthetic and a small amount of opiate. The sedative effects of epidural opiates may last up to 24 hours after the epidural infusion has stopped, and will be additive to the sedative effects of other drugs. The side-effects of opiate medications can be very troublesome, and include delirium, confusion, withdrawal syndromes, pruritus, constipation, nausea and vomiting. As well as providing pain relief, opiates also have the useful effect of suppressing respiratory drive in patients who are unable to synchronise respiratory effort with a ventilator.

Systemic opiates are often given as a continuous infusion. *Morphine* is commonly used in this way on the ICU, but has the disadvantage of possessing a prolonged effect. In addition, the presence of liver or renal failure may exaggerate its actions, allowing it to persist in the circulation long after administration has ceased. For this reason, many ICUs have moved to using infusions of shorter-acting but more powerful opiates, such as *fentanyl*, *alfentanil* and *remifentanil*. These drugs are synthetic opiates that are similar in chemical structure to *pethidine*. They are many times more powerful than morphine. *Sufentanil* is used in some countries, but is not licensed in the UK.

Remifentanil in particular is being used with increasing frequency on the ICU, as it is metabolised spontaneously in the bloodstream, and is therefore not dependent on liver metabolism or renal excretion. It is very potent, but its duration of action is very short. If the syringe of remifentanil that is being infused to the patient runs out, there will not be time to mix up the next syringe before the effects of the first one start to wear off. It is therefore recommended that the nursing staff have the next syringe of remifentanil prepared and ready to use well in advance. As this drug is very potent, it is increasingly being used as the sole means of sedation in some cases. However, it is not yet recommended that this is tried outside of the ICU, as the therapeutic window is quite small. Remifentanil is also not recommended for use by non-anaesthetists. However, many authorities believe that utilising remifentanil as the sole analgesic/sedative agent (so-called *analgesic sedation*) results in a more comfortable, more cooperative ICU patient.

Newer agents which act peripherally as opiate antagonists, such as alvimopan and methylnaltrexone, are thought to reduce the incidence of opiate-induced problems without depreciating the analgesic effects, and may become increasingly used in the future in conjunction with opiate infusions.

Studies have shown that the analgesic requirements of ICU patients may be underestimated by staff. This is mainly because of communication difficulties. The regular use of assessment tools, such as the Behavioural Pain Scale, has been shown to improve patient comfort.[2] Such scales utilise an objective assessment of patient characteristics (e.g. facial expression) and assign a score to each parameter. A high score might be taken to indicate poor analgesia, and the dose of painkiller would then be increased. It would be expected that medical staff would prescribe a dose range for the opiate infusion, with an instruction to vary the rate within that range in order to keep the pain score below a set level. A typical pain score is shown in Table 11.2.[3]

TABLE 11.2 A typical ICU pain score

PARAMETER	1	2	3	4
Facial expression	Relaxed	Partially tightened	Fully tightened	Grimacing
Upper limb movements	None	Partially bent	Fully bent with finger flexion	Permanently retracted
Compliance with mechanical ventilation	Tolerating movement	Coughing but tolerating movement most of the time	Fighting ventilator	Unable to control ventilation

Analgesia can be increased in anticipation of patient requirements. For example, if the patient is to undergo an invasive procedure, it is sensible to anticipate pain by administering a pre-emptive bolus dose of painkiller. Non-sedating analgesics, such as paracetamol, given regularly are useful adjuncts in lowering the total amount of opiate that needs to be administered over the course of the patient's stay.

It is now regarded as best practice to address the patient's analgesic needs as the first priority, and then to introduce sedative drugs as required.[4]

Sedation

Sedation on the ICU will be utilised for three main purposes, namely to allow toleration of ongoing treatment, to reduce agitation and discomfort, and to allow 'one-off' interventions (e.g. line insertion). While they are heavily sedated, patients may be receiving treatment from complex devices, such as haemofilters, but will still require basic care for personal and hygiene needs.

The commonest mode of sedation on the ICU involves the use of continuous drug infusion with either propofol or midazolam. Propofol can be administered as a 1% or 2% solution, and midazolam is usually administered at a concentration of 2 or 5 mg/ml. Both agents have advantages and drawbacks.

Propofol is a general anaesthetic agent which has a rapid onset and offset, and its effects are easily titrated against the patient's response. However, the lipid solution carrier agent provides a high calorific load, and there have been cases of hyperlipidaemia and fatty liver reported after prolonged administration. Propofol is no longer routinely used in paediatric ICUs, following deaths associated with fatty liver, acidosis and cardiomyopathy. There have been recent reports of this so-called *propofol infusion syndrome* occurring in adults.[5] Midazolam can also be titrated to effect. However, it may take longer than expected to wear off, perhaps prolonging ventilation and ultimately the ICU stay, particularly in the elderly. Tolerance to both drugs may develop very quickly, leading to an increased rate or concentration of infusion with little therapeutic benefit. For this reason, many ICUs will rotate the sedative drugs that they use, occasionally utilising agents other than those already described.

Infusions of *thiopentone* (a general anaesthetic barbiturate) are occasionally used, but cause histamine release and metabolic alkalosis. *Ketamine* is sometimes utilised, particularly in patients with severe asthma, where its bronchodilatory effect can be very beneficial, but it can be associated with acidosis and violent hallucinations. *Etomidate* is no longer used in ICU practice, as it is associated with hypothalamic axis depression and increased mortality. Newer drugs such as *dexmedetomidine* may become available for widespread use in the future. This drug has both analgesic and sedative effects, and may have a less depressant effect on the cardiovascular system.

The practice of ICU sedation

An infused drug with a starting concentration in the patient of 0 mg/ml will take 4 half-lives to achieve a steady-state concentration in the plasma. This means that considerable time elapses before the patient may be properly sedated. It is therefore usual either to give the patient an initial bolus of sedative/anaesthetic drug before the infusion is started, or to start the sedation infusion at a much higher rate than is initially required, and to reduce the rate of infusion later.

Although an ICU patient may initially need to be anaesthetised on admission, when undergoing active, invasive treatment and procedures, once their condition is stable, attempts must begin to bring down the level of sedation required. This may involve the addition of regular oral/nasogastric sedation such as lorazepam to the patient's treatment regime, or the introduction of drugs with novel sedative effects, such as clonidine. The patient should remain comfortable and anxiety-free, but if sedation is too light, they may become distressed and uncooperative, resulting in difficulties in treatment.

The routine use of a *sedation score* can greatly assist the management of ICU patients. This was first proposed as a standard practice in the UK by the Intensive Care Society.[6,7] A typical score is shown in Table 11.3.

TABLE 11.3 A simplified ICU sedation score

HOURLY SCORE	3	2	1	0	−1	−2	−3
Definition	Agitated and restless	Awake and uncomfortable	Awake but calm and comfortable	Roused by voice	Roused by touch	Roused by painful stimuli	Cannot be roused

Such simple scores can easily be accommodated into local clinical guidelines. Instruction can be given to review the sedation score at set intervals, and then to vary the rate of sedation by a set amount to achieve a set score. It could be standard practice to assume that most patients should be kept at a level of 0 to 1 unless other instructions are given.

A second recommended method of assessing the sedation requirement is that of *sedation breaks.* This suggests that the sedation should be completely stopped at least once a day, and the patient should be allowed to wake up completely. If the patient is uncooperative or agitated, sedation can be restarted. This method may be particularly useful if the patient has been deeply rather than lightly sedated, and it enables staff to perform a neurological assessment and to determine sedation and analgesic requirements. However, it can also be argued that such a system exposes the patient unnecessarily to the risks of pain and anxiety.

Muscle relaxants

It should be noted that, on occasion, ICU patients may also be receiving muscle relaxant drugs, such as atracurium, particularly if the use of sedation and analgesia has not adequately allowed safe mechanical ventilation to occur. A patient who is paralysed will of course be completely unresponsive to outside stimuli, and it is therefore possible that they may be paralysed but *not* sedated, a situation akin to being 'awake under an anaesthetic' or 'locked in.' Therefore the muscle-paralysing agent should be stopped at regular intervals to allow the sedation level to be properly assessed.

Important considerations with regard to sedation on the ICU are shown in Table 11.4.

TABLE 11.4 Important considerations with regard to sedation on the ICU[7]

All patients must be comfortable and pain-free. Analgesia is the first aim.
Anxiety should be minimised. This is difficult, as anxiety is an appropriate emotion. The most important way of achieving this is to provide compassionate and considerate care. Communication is an essential part of this.
Patients should be calm, cooperative and able to sleep when undisturbed. This does not mean that they must be asleep at all times.
Patients must be able to tolerate appropriate organ system support. This is particularly important in patients who require complex mechanical ventilatory patterns, or permissive hypercapnia. If it is impossible to ensure synchronisation of the patient's own respiratory effort with the ventilator without risk of sedative overdose, there may be a need for neuromuscular blockade. The use of a nerve stimulator to monitor the extent of neuromuscular blockade may be useful in some situations.
Patients must not be paralysed and awake. Remember to stop muscle relaxant in order to check the sedation level.
Any avoidable source of physical discomfort should be anticipated, identified and treated.
The need for any uncomfortable or disturbing therapies should be minimised.
A perceived need to increase sedatives may be an index of clinical deterioration.
When sedation has been stopped, night sleep is often fitful because of rebound REM sleep.
Continued night sedation may prolong this disturbing phenomenon, rather than treat it.
Non-drug measures (e.g. massage, etc.) should be considered.

Complications of sedation on the ICU

Many of the common complications of sedation on ICU are related to the patient's altered physiology, and are often exaggerated known side-effects (e.g. excessive hypotension, bradycardia, prolonged action, etc.). Sometimes, increasing doses are required as the patient develops tolerance of the drugs used. Some medications, like propofol and etomidate, are known to be associated with specific fatal complications (see above).

Physically, the longer a patient stays sedated on the ICU the more likely they are to acquire complications such as lung atelectasis, secondary infections, thrombotic events and even pressure sores due to their relative immobility. Patients who have prolonged stays may also develop muscle wasting and weakness, the so-called *ICU myopathy/neuropathy* syndromes.

Prolonged use of sedatives can have profound psychological effects on patients. The ICU staff should always be aware that the sudden cessation of infusions that the patient has been receiving for some time may result in a withdrawal syndrome. This is possible with opiates and benzodiazepines, and can also occur in relation to drugs that the patient was consuming before they became critically ill (e.g. alcohol, nicotine). Some patients may require a phased reduction in sedation as a result, or substitution of the intravenous sedative/opiate infusion with another oral drug while they are recovering.

Sedatives themselves alter the patient's perception of events and their surroundings. Although some drugs, such as ketamine, are known to cause hallucinations, simple misinterpretation of everyday ICU events by sedated patients due to their impaired consciousness has been associated with a kind of post-traumatic stress syndrome, commonly known as 'ICU psychosis.' The effects vary, but they can include anxiety, panic attacks, flashbacks and hallucinations. Patients may be convinced that bizarre and threatening things were happening, and may believe that staff were trying to harm them. Distortions of memory can also occur because of amnesia induced by midazolam.

Proper management of sedation control is associated with a reduction in the incidence of this problem. However, staff should be aware of the signs and symptoms of confusion and delirium.[8,9] Proper communication with patients is essential, and keeping an ICU diary for each patient may well put into context events that they recall later when they are physically well. In addition, the early administration of antidepressants should be considered for patients who will have prolonged stays. Antipsychotic drugs may be required to treat agitation due to hallucinations.[10–12]

Summary

The sedation of patients on the ICU is a specialist field which aims to reduce anxiety in critically ill patients who are undergoing active, invasive treatment. Complications can arise due to the altered physiology of the patients, and also due to the average length of time for which patients are usually subject to analgesic and sedative infusions. Best practice, involving the use of sedation and analgesic scores and regular assessment of patient needs, can reduce complications and aid patient recovery.

LEARNING POINTS

- The practice of sedation on the ICU is similar to the practice of total intravenous anaesthesia (TIVA). This may be used in combination with other oral sedatives. The patient's analgesic requirements must be met. The administration of muscle relaxants may be necessary, but these drugs should be used with caution.
- The sedation should be prescribed by doctors and managed by nurses according to a local guideline, incorporating a targeted sedation score.
- Sedation scores or sedation breaks are a necessary part of the treatment plan to reduce the incidence of over-sedation, prolonged stays and sedation-related complications.
- Prolonged use of sedation can have adverse side-effects.

References

1 Department of Health. *Comprehensive Critical Care*; http://www.ics.ac.uk/downloads/ICM%20Prof_Pulications_Other%20publications/Other%20organisation%20and%20NHS%20publications%20below/Comprehensive%20Critical%20Care.pdf (accessed 9 August 2007).

2 Assaoui Y, Zeggwagh AA, Zekraoui A *et al.* Validation of a behavioural pain scale in critically ill, sedated and mechanically ventilated patients. *Anesth Analg.* 2005; **101:** 1470–6.

3 Payen JF, Bru O, Bosson JL *et al.* Assessing pain in critically ill sedated patients by using a behavioural pain scale. *Crit Care Med.* 2001; **29:** 2258–63.

4 Fraser GL, Riker R. Sedation and analgesia in the critically ill adult. *Curr Opin Anaesthesiol.* 2007; **20:** 119–23.

5 Kam PLA, Cardone D. Propofol infusion syndrome. *Anaesthesia.* 2007; **82:** 690–701.

6 Rosser D, Saich C, Buckley R *et al. Intensive Care Society National Guidelines. Sedation Guideline.* London: Intensive Care Society; 1999.

7 Intensive Care Society. *Clinical Standards Committee. Sedation Guideline*; www.ics.ac.uk/icmprof/downloads/sedation.pdf (accessed 31 May 2007).

8 Devlin JW, Fong JJ, Fraser GL *et al.* Delirium assessment in the critically ill. *Intensive Care Med.* 2007; **33:** 929–40.

9 Ebersoldt M, Sharshar T, Annane D. Sepsis-associated delirium. *Intensive Care Med.* 2007; **33:** 941–50.

10 Borthwick M, Bourne R, Craig M *et al. Detection, Prevention and Treatment of Delirium in Critically Ill Patients.* South Wigston: United Kingdom Clinical Pharmacy Association; 2006.

11 Griffiths RD, Jones C. Delirium, cognitive dysfunction and post-traumatic stress disorder. *Curr Opin Anaesthesiol.* 2007; **20:** 124–9.

12 Ridley S, editor. *Critical Care Focus 12. The psychological challenges of intensive care.* London: BMJ Books; 2005.

CHAPTER 12

Sedation in palliative care

'Palliative care' is the term used to define a treatment programme that aims to provide comfort and dignity for those believed to be in the process of dying, and is now recognised in the UK as a distinct medical field that requires specialist training and expertise. A holistic approach to the patient is advocated, in order to ensure that social, family and spiritual needs are all addressed with the same urgency as physical symptoms. Such treatment programmes can include alleviation of distressing manifestations such as pain, breathlessness, thirst, nutritional problems and delirium. Appropriate use of sedation may be an important part of such a treatment plan, but may impair the ability of the patient to express their wishes, particularly if the sedative acts synergistically with other drugs, such as opiates. If the interests of the dying patient are to remain paramount, it is important that the treatment plan is reviewed regularly and proactively with the patient.

The practice of palliative sedation

Various definitions of 'palliative sedation' have been suggested, but the common goal is to reduce intractable physical and existential distress, up to the point of inducing and maintaining a deep sleep, but not deliberately causing death.[1] However, it is possible that the treatment itself may have the unintended consequence of hastening the patient's inevitable demise. This is the so-called 'double (or dual) effect', which was first enshrined in British law in the infamous Bodkin Adams case.[2,3] This doctrine can be summarised as follows:

The duty of the doctor or nurse is to relieve suffering, and it is permissible to administer drugs in order to achieve this; however, a patient at the end of their life, who is suffering greatly, may require such large drug doses to preserve their comfort and dignity that the possible side-effects of these drugs (such as respiratory depression) may *incidentally* accelerate the act of dying.

In other words, if the consequence of not administering the drug is that the patient would continue to suffer up to the imminent and inevitable point of death, the doctor has a duty to do all that they can to relieve that suffering, so long as they do not *intentionally* act to end the patient's life (*see* Box 12.1).

BOX 12.1 Legal clarification of the double effect doctrine

Mrs L was diagnosed with motor neuron disease. As her illness progressed, she became aware that the terminal stages of the illness could be associated with very distressing symptoms. She launched a legal attempt to obtain a High Court Order to force her doctors to give her diamorphine in quantities which would deliberately shorten her life. The case was abandoned when it was reiterated that it was lawful for doctors to administer analgesics and sedatives in these circumstances, even if death might be hastened, provided that the *intent* was to relieve suffering, not to kill.

Lords Hansard text for 20 November 1997. *Terminally Ill Patients*; www. parliament.the-stationery-office.co.uk/pa/ld199798/ldhansrd/vo971120/ text/71120-20.htm (accessed 13 July 2007).

Administration of a drug with the express intention of ending the patient's life is termed *euthanasia*, and although this is legal in some countries, is still against the law in the UK.

Patients with a fatal prognosis may be fearful of a loss of autonomy, and anxious that value decisions will be made about their treatment when they are no longer able to represent themselves.[4] Medical and nursing staff must ensure that such patients are counselled from an appropriate stage, so that they can ensure that their wishes are expressed in an appropriate form, such as a living will, or a lasting power of attorney (LPA).

The use of palliative sedation may not always indicate that death is imminent. For example, it is possible that the administration of sedation for a brief period to a patient suffering from a terminal condition may relieve distressing symptoms. Some authorities have attempted to define different stages of sedation for terminally ill patients. These stages range from increasing the dose of sedative drugs that the patient is already prescribed, to continual infusion of sedatives, and they are defined in Table 12.1.

TABLE 12.1 Defined stages of terminal sedation

Routine sedation	Introduction of normal doses of sedative medication, or an increase in the doses of sedative drugs that the patient is already receiving, in order to alleviate symptoms (e.g. insomnia, anxiety, etc.).
Infrequent sedation	Upward titration of drugs used for routine sedation, and conversion of essential medications to non-oral administration routes as symptoms become more severe.
Extraordinary sedation	Continuous infusion of drugs for the relief of symptoms in the dying and those who are unable to continue to take sedation in the normal manner.

Although death can occur at any time in the terminally ill, it is the introduction of *extraordinary sedation* (also known as *terminal sedation*) that has the greatest chance of accelerating an impending death. It is clear, therefore, that a degree of medico-legal preparation may be required before extraordinary sedation can be administered. The recommended pre-conditions are listed in Table 12.2.

TABLE 12.2 Pre-conditions for the use of extraordinary sedation in terminally ill patients

The illness is documented as irreversible, and death is imminent (within hours or days).
The symptoms that require relief are well defined and understood, and unbearable to the patient.
A palliative care expert has been consulted and is in agreement that extraordinary sedation is appropriate.
Informed consent has been obtained from the patient. The patient must be fully informed about their condition, and must have been given a chance to express their own wishes. The relatives have been counselled, and they understand and accept the treatment plan.
A proper plan for the prescription and use of sedation has been fully documented. This will include whether the sedation is to be continuous or intermittent, under what circumstances it may be increased or decreased, and which side-effects are to be treated.
Contraindications to sedation or to the proposed medications have been confirmed as absent. Patient refusal is a contraindication.

cont.

As the patient's condition is terminal, and as death is expected to be imminent, a 'Do Not Attempt Resuscitation' (DNAR) order has been documented, and has been communicated to all staff.

All staff dealing with the patient fully understand the treatment that has been initiated.

Plans to maintain the basic healthcare needs of the patient are in place. This will include pressure area care, mouth care, catheter care, etc.

When a patient is terminally ill, and suffering, it is possible that drugs are used in excessive doses to alleviate that suffering, or that medications normally used for other purposes are utilised in novel ways. Although staff may come under intense psychological pressure to relieve very distressing symptoms, they must ensure that they continue to practise within ethical and legal boundaries (*see* Box 12.2).

BOX 12.2 Straying outside legal boundaries in terminal care

Mrs B was a terminally ill patient who was in great distress. Her pain and suffering were so great that she repeatedly begged for her life to be ended. Standard medication such as morphine was ineffective. Dr C, a rheumatology consultant, administered intravenous potassium chloride to Mrs B, who died soon afterwards. Dr C was found guilty of attempted murder, and received a suspended sentence. He also received a reprimand from the GMC. During the trial, the judge specifically instructed the jury to decide whether the doctor's primary intent was to kill, and to disregard his possible motives in administering the injection, and the patient's repeated requests for euthanasia.

R v Cox [1992] 12v BMLR 38.
Euthanasia: an overview; http://news.bbc.co.uk/1/health/background_briefings/euthanasia/331255.stm

Case histories: end-of-life decisions; http://news.bbc.co.uk/1/hi/programmes/1971527.stm
(Both websites accessed 13 July 2007)

Neuromuscular blocking agents

In recent years there has been some discussion in the medical literature of the use of muscle relaxants (neuromuscular blocking agents) in terminal care. The specific circumstances in this debate concern the removal of terminally ill neonates from a ventilator in order to allow them to die in the arms of their parents, a time at which terminal, spasmodic breathing attempts can occur. Anaesthetic muscle relaxants have been suggested as a way of preventing these 'agonal breaths.' Medical opinion is divided as to the appropriateness of this suggestion. Opponents of the idea suggest that because the sole purpose of such a muscle relaxant is to paralyse the patient in order to facilitate mechanical ventilation, and since ventilation is not instituted the patient will die from hypoxia, the dual effect cannot therefore apply – the doctor has acted to end the life of the patient. Proponents argue that such patients have been withdrawn from invasive treatment, and are in the act of dying anyway, and that as the intent of administering the muscle relaxant is to relieve distress, the dual effect doctrine is valid. Neither of these positions has yet been tested in law, but they have been tested by the UK medical regulatory body, the General Medical Council (*see* Box 12.3).[5–8]

BOX 12.3 Muscle relaxants used for the treatment of agonal respiration

It was discovered that Dr M had given large doses of the muscle relaxant pancuronium to two terminally ill children after removing them from ventilators. Active medical treatment had been withdrawn on the grounds of futility, and the children were suffering agonal gasping which had not responded to opiates. Dr M had explained to both parents that the process of dying was taking much longer than anticipated, and in both cases obtained their agreement to give the paralysing agent, acknowledging that it was on the boundary of what society regarded as acceptable. Dr M was referred to the GMC, where he was found not guilty of serious professional misconduct. The GMC acknowledged that medical opinion in this area was contradictory, that no guidelines existed, and that Dr M had acted primarily to relieve suffering.

Urquhart F. Doctor gave 23 times the normal dose of drug to dying babies; http://thescotsman.scotsman.com/index.cfm?id=1053952007

Baby death panel dismisses claim; http://news.bbc.co.uk/1/hi/scotland/north_east/6289686

Doctor cleared over fatal baby injections; http://society.guardian.co.uk/health/story/0,,2123766,00.html?gusrc==rss&feed==network
(All websites accessed 12 July 2007)

Summary

Sedation can form a valid and important part of a treatment programme for terminally ill patients. However, such a course of action should not be entered into lightly, and involves a high degree of trust and partnership between the healthcare staff, the patient and the patient's relatives. It should be utilised only within a strict clinical governance framework that has been agreed by the multi-disciplinary team managing the patient.

LEARNING POINTS

- Sedation in palliative care is a specialist field.
- The medico-legal framework governing this field of practice is complex.
- It should be clear that the purpose of sedation in these circumstances is to relieve suffering, not to bring about death.

References

1 Vissers KCP, Hasselaar J, Verhagen SAHHVM. Sedation in palliative care. *Curr Opin Anaesthesiol.* 2007; **20:** 137–42.
2 *R v Adams* [1957] Crim LR 3.
3 Cullen PV. *A Stranger in Blood. The case files on Dr John Bodkin Adams.* London: Elliot & Thompson; 2007.
4 *R (Burke) v General Medical Council* [2004] 79 BMLR.
5 Hatherill M, Tibby SM, Sykes K *et al.* Dilemmas exist in withdrawing ventilation from dying children. *BMJ.* 1998; **317:** 80.
6 Perkin RM, Resnik DB. The agony of agonal respiration: is the last gasp necessary? *J Med Ethics.* 2002; **28:** 134–69.
7 Street K, Henderson J. The distinction between withdrawing life-sustaining treatment under the influence of paralysing agents and euthanasia. *BMJ.* 2001; **323:** 388–91.
8 Soloman MZ, Sellers DE, Heller KS *et al.* New and lingering controversies in paediatric end-of-life care. *Paediatrics.* 2005; **116:** 872–83.

CHAPTER 13

Sedation for miscellaneous procedures

Sedation is given to assist the performance of numerous procedures, many of which will require no more than the application of the basic principles of safe practice already described. However, there are some circumstances in which the practicalities of the proposed procedure or investigation are sufficiently different to warrant specific discussion. The aim of this chapter is to briefly outline the main considerations for some of the more common of these miscellaneous activities which present unique challenges for the sedationist. It is worth remembering that the low mortality and morbidity associated with many of these interventions may be more related to the brevity of their duration than to the inherent safety of the technique, and the sedationist should ensure that they never take their responsibility to the patient lightly just because the complication rate is perceived to be low.

Assorted medical procedures

Bronchoscopy

Direct bronchoscopy is used in the investigation of serious airway symptoms, particularly when cancer is suspected. Patients are often elderly, and may have multiple pathologies in addition to their lung disease. The nasal passages are prepared with a mixture of local anaesthetic and vasoconstrictor, which not only provides analgesia, but also reduces the possibility of bleeding caused by the trauma of passing the fibre-optic bronchoscope. The nostril to be utilised must be chosen with care, as problems such as a deviated septum or nasal polyps can lead to pain and bleeding. The patient is usually positioned sitting upright, with the bronchoscopist standing to their front at one side. The back of the throat is anaesthetised with local anaesthetic spray, oxygen is administered (often through nasal specula) and the scope is inserted. Local anaesthetic is sprayed under direct vision on to pharyngeal and laryngeal structures through the scope as it is passed. Sedation is often required, because the local anaesthetic does not completely eliminate unpleasant gagging or coughing. The procedure can take a variable length of time depending upon the degree of difficulty and operator experience. The patient is usually monitored by means of a pulse oximeter.

Anaesthetists sometimes use a similar technique, termed *awake intubation*, when they need to insert an endotracheal tube for surgery, but do not wish to render the patient unconscious first (e.g. in the case of a patient with an unstable neck). A variety of techniques have been described, ranging from the 'spray local as you go' approach to the administration of specific nerve blocks in the neck. Sedation is sometimes used in these circumstances, although airway compromise is a concern.

Cardioversion

Cardioversion is the use of an electric shock to convert a cardiac arrhythmia (commonly atrial fibrillation) back into a sinus rhythm. In principle, this is no different to defibrillation in cardiac arrest, except that the patient still has a cardiac output and so is likely to be conscious, and a much smaller shock is used. The shock must be synchronised with the ECG morphology so that the risk of inducing an arrest rhythm is minimised. Cardioversion can be performed as an emergency or as an elective procedure. The usual indications for emergency cardioversion are that the patient's condition is unstable and drug therapy has failed. In elective cases, the patient's condition is stable with the arrhythmia, but a return to sinus rhythm is required to reduce the risk of embolic stroke and other conditions that can result. Such patients are usually anti-coagulated.

Sedation is required for this procedure because of the high level of pre-existing patient anxiety, and for the management of the peri- and post-shock pain that can result. Many units utilise anaesthetists for this process, who commonly administer propofol or etomidate to induce a brief period of anaesthesia. However, several units now utilise a nurse-led sedation protocol for this procedure,[1] which has been shown to have low complication rates. Local protocols may vary according to the type of defibrillator used or the number of shocks given. Common difficulties include failure to convert the rhythm (in which case repeat shocks may be required), or hypotension after successful conversion. The use of sedation itself can of course induce low blood pressure. It has therefore been recommended that all patients should receive full monitoring.[2]

The patient may suffer painful burns to the chest due to excessive shock or poorly placed paddles. It is also possible for the shock to arc across the chest if the patient is sweaty, or if too much contact gel is used. Staff should stand clear of the patient trolley, and oxygen should be removed from the patient when the shock is being administered.

Gastroscopy and colonoscopy

Traditionally, sedation for endoscopic procedures is provided by the endoscopist, typically using midazolam, either alone or in combination with an opiate, usually pethidine. The oropharyngeal gag reflex is often abolished using local anaesthetic spray. This will result in the patient being unable to swallow properly for some time, so one of the discharge criteria should be that normal swallowing function has returned.

Side-effects such as nausea and vomiting are common following upper gastrointestinal endoscopy, and recent National Confidential Enquiry into Patient Outcome and Death (NCEPOD) guidance in the UK[3] has focused attention on the use of other agents, such as propofol. The use of propofol has caused controversy in the USA, where the Anaesthetic and Gastroenterological Societies have produced different guidance as to who should administer it.[4,5] In America, approximately 25% of endoscopies are performed using propofol-based deep sedation (i.e. anaesthesia).[6] The incidence of cases where it is necessary to rescue the patient with bag and mask ventilation appears to be low. Patient-controlled sedation has been used in some cases, but appears to be associated with a variable level of success. Target-controlled sedation using infusions of propofol may be a better alternative, but the safety profile of this technique when utilised by non-anaesthetists has not been defined.

Lower bowel endoscopy often requires a degree of preparation with powerful laxative medication. This may dehydrate the patient, and can result in hypotension on induction of sedation, particularly in the elderly.

Endoscopy is also performed in emergency situations, commonly in patients who are suffering from a gastrointestinal bleed. It is possible that even if the bleeding has stopped, the stomach may be full of blood, so that aspiration due to a reduction in protective reflexes is a possibility when sedation is induced. The patient may also be in shock, so the hypotensive effects of sedation may be exaggerated. In such cases it is recommended that intravenous access is secured with a large-bore cannula, so that resuscitation fluid can be administered briskly in the event of an emergency.

Anaesthesia might perhaps be a better alternative for some patients in these circumstances.

Endoscopic retrograde cholangiopancreatography (ERCP) can be used to treat a variety of conditions, particularly gallstone disease, and can be performed safely under sedation. However, pancreatitis can result following instrumental manipulation of the biliary tree.

It has been recommended that all patients who are undergoing endoscopy under sedation should have a proper intravenous cannula *in situ*, receive supplementary oxygen, and have at least ECG and pulse oximetry monitored. It is recommended that no patient should be so sedated with benzodiazepine as to require reversal with flumazenil, and that the procedure failure rate due to inadequate sedation should be less than 5%.[7]

Electroconvulsive therapy (ECT)

ECT is a rare (and possibly the only) example of a sedation technique including muscle relaxant. In essence, it is believed that the administration of an electric shock to the brain is an effective treatment for severe depression, as the current alters the level of neurotransmitters. There is continuing debate about the effectiveness of the treatment, but there is general agreement that the resulting convulsions need to be modified using muscle relaxants in order to prevent injury to the patient from muscle spasms. Commonly the patient is rendered unconscious using a reduced, titrated dose of either barbiturate or propofol (or possibly a propofol infusion) and a much reduced dose of suxamethonium given intravenously. Suxamethonium is a depolarising anaesthetic muscle relaxant which quickly induces flaccid paralysis, stopping breathing, but thereby reducing the severity of the convulsion. It is therefore necessary to support the airway until normal respiration recommences. In normal circumstances, the muscle relaxation effects wear off very quickly. However, in susceptible individuals, particularly those who lack the enzyme that metabolises suxamethonium, a considerable period of time can elapse before spontaneous respiration occurs (so-called *scoline apnoea*). Therefore, although there are some instances where the 'anaesthetic' is given by non-anaesthetists,[8] the common situation is that it is a qualified anaesthetist who administers the drugs and cares for the patient. It should be remembered that although such patients may well be physically fit, they will be subject to the administration of powerful psychoactive drugs with many side-effects and interactions. In addition, there have been many concerns raised over the years about the standard of the facilities within which such procedures are performed.[9,10]

Surgical procedures

Anaesthetists continually assert that there is no such thing as a 'quick general anaesthetic', because a general anaesthetic for a short surgical procedure requires exactly the same safety considerations and preparation as that for a longer one. This simple maxim also applies to the use of sedation. Many minor surgical procedures can be performed under a combination of local anaesthesia and sedation, or sedation alone. On occasion, this may be under the control of an operator-sedationist. However, the same safety practices apply to these situations as to any other in which sedation is utilised.

Emergency department

Patients with less urgent conditions that require treatment under sedation may be able to return later in the day to a dedicated casualty clinic. This clinic should be properly staffed, and must satisfy the same equipment and safety criteria as any other area where sedation is performed. In general, such patients are presenting electively, and should be prepared and recovered as if they are undergoing day-case anaesthesia, although there is still some controversy as to whether full starvation restrictions should apply to all patients.

This work should only be performed by those who are specifically trained. It should not be delegated to the occasional practitioner.

Immediate treatment is necessary for life- or limb-threatening conditions which could result in serious harm or disablement. In addition, there are some less serious conditions which, if dealt with swiftly, can obviate the need for more complex intervention later on. These can include procedures such as manipulation of fractures or the treatment of dislocated shoulders. Although it may be extremely tempting to subject someone to a 'quick' procedure in the casualty department on these grounds, this should not be at the risk of unnecessary hazard to the patient, or merely for the convenience of the surgeon.

Departments should have a local policy in place to deal with these situations, which should define how the patients are sedated, in what location, and by whom, and – equally importantly – how the patient is recovered, and when and to where they can be discharged. Emergency departments should not therefore allow staff from other specialties to administer sedation to patients on their premises without proper planning and supervision. Although in some circumstances there may be no option but to proceed as quickly as possible, if there is any doubt about the safety of a procedure, there should be a low threshold for taking the patient immediately to theatre and proceeding under proper anaesthetic cover with minimum delay.

Possible hazards include patients having a full stomach or being under the influence of alcohol (both of which predispose to aspiration), the unpredictable effect of drugs in emergency situations, interactions occurring with other drugs that the patient may have ingested, deterioration in the patient's coexisting medical conditions, and the risks related to the presence of a sedationist-operator – a role which may be unavoidable under emergency circumstances.

General surgical, urological and orthopaedic practice

Procedures commonly performed under sedation include endoscopic examinations, the drainage of abscesses, and the removal of simple lumps or growths. Usually these operations have been arranged as elective procedures. It is essential that patients have been subject to a rigorous selection process, especially if the operating list is being performed without the presence of an anaesthetist. A situation where the operator-sedationist is at the critical point of the procedure and the patient is in distress is a disaster, as is the scenario where the patient succumbs to over-sedation halfway through the procedure. If there is any doubt at any stage about the ability to perform the procedure under sedation as planned, anaesthetic opinion or assistance should be sought. The performance of surgical procedures under sedation should be subjected to rigorous audit in order to ensure that practice remains acceptable.

Gynaecological and obstetric practice

As in general surgical practice, many gynaecological procedures can be performed under sedation, but often a general anaesthetic is preferred by the patient.

Pregnant patients may also require minor procedures and investigations to be performed, which might require the use of sedation, but there are many considerations that the sedationist must bear in mind. The physiology of the pregnant woman is significantly different to that of the non-pregnant female. As pregnancy progresses, airway anatomy may alter, resulting in a higher incidence of airway management problems in the event of over-sedation. Furthermore, the presence of an abdominal mass (the fetus) and hormonal changes result in an increased incidence of gastric reflux, and consequent risk of aspiration. Cardiac output is higher, and blood pressure is generally lower. Early in pregnancy, sedationists must be careful to use drugs that are not associated with teratogenicity in the fetus. Later in pregnancy, they must consider the fact that sedatives might cross the placenta and accumulate in the baby (resulting in respiratory depression if parturition occurs soon afterwards) or cross into the newborn through breast milk. In addition, obstetric patients can suffer from illnesses that are specific to pregnancy, such as severe vomiting or pre-eclampsia, which will require expert advice.

Otolaryngology (ear, nose and throat)

In general, anaesthesia is preferred to facilitate investigations and minor operations in ENT practice, although some relatively non-invasive procedures (such as nasal endoscopy or flexible bronchoscopy) can be performed under sedation. The considerations in relation to sedation for this are similar to those for dental practice, in that the sedationist will share responsibility for the airway with the surgeon.

Ophthalmology[11]

Over the last decade there has been a revolution in ophthalmic surgical practice. Due to improved surgical techniques and technology, in particular the increased use of phaeco-emulsification, many operations which were performed almost exclusively under general anaesthetic are now being offered as day-case surgery under local anaesthesia with or without sedation. In addition, local anaesthetic techniques have improved, reducing inconvenience, pain and anxiety for the patient. In particular, straightforward cataract surgery can now be performed under topical local anaesthetic in most cases, avoiding altogether the inconvenience and discomfort of the several injections to the face and orbit that previous techniques necessitated.

The main consideration is that the surgeon requires a very cooperative patient. In particular, the patient must be able to lie flat for a short period of time (20 to 30 minutes), and must be able to keep the eyeball and head still during surgery. This requires good pre-operative preparation and counselling, which must ensure that the patient knows exactly what sensations they may experience. It is also important to remember that during the procedure the patient will be completely isolated. The face and head will often be covered by a sterile sheet, which can impair hearing as well as vision. Often the support of someone holding the patient's hand is reassuring and can prevent the need for further intervention. Anxiety can be countered effectively by continuity of staffing, reassurance and constructive discussion with the rest of the surgical team. For example, if a patient feels claustrophobic, the surgeon may be able to make some useful accommodation by altering the position of the sterile sheeting. However, there may well be a valid medical reason why the patient cannot have their surgery under local anaesthetic alone (e.g. a neurological condition such as Parkinson's disease may prevent the patient from lying still). Such conditions should be identified early in the pre-operative assessment phase.

If sedation is considered to be a necessary adjunct to local anaesthetic, serious consideration should be given to whether a general anaesthetic is an appropriate intervention, as it will more reliably reproduce the ophthalmic conditions that the surgeon requires. It is thought that less than 10% of patients should require sedation for cataract surgery. The aim as always is to reduce anxiety while maintaining safety. This is all the more important in view of the fact that many ophthalmic patients are elderly, and may have multiple coexisting disease states, as a result of which they are subject to polypharmacy. Therefore sedation should be provided in a planned manner by competent sedationists. Sedation should not be used to compensate for an inadequate local block. A very light level of sedation to reduce anxiety is all that is necessary. A recent paper has suggested that the use of topical anaesthesia in combination with oral sedation was a safe combination, to the extent that an anaesthetist did not need to be present in theatre.[12] It should be noted that this paper did find an incidence of 15.6 % for adverse events, the majority of which were dealt with successfully by the surgeon. However, the overall incidence of serious events that required anaesthetic intervention was 0.9%. The authors also controversially suggested that the safety of this technique meant that the usual pre-operative examination and investigations were not required.

All patients should receive oxygen-enriched air for the duration of the procedure, and this can be administered in a variety of ways. However, a face mask or nasal specula may interfere with the surgical field. Often the oxygen is administered through a pipe into a box which sits under the sterile sheeting on the patient's chest, turning the sterile sheeting into a kind of oxygen tent. The type of monitoring that should be utilised during eye surgery under local anaesthesia is debatable. Many experts argue that the use of a self-inflating blood pressure cuff can disturb the patient sufficiently to cause undesirable movement during surgery, and so will dispense with its use in routine cases. Others suggest that the use of a pulse oximeter which displays a pulse trace as well as a saturation reading is safe for the majority of cases, and that full monitoring is only necessary for those at serious risk of complications. However, it is recommended that the standard of monitoring utilised for patients who are receiving sedation should be similar to that used during general anaesthesia, although use of an ECG may depend on the requirements of the sedationist. Whatever monitoring is used, the sedationist should be aware that they would be expected to justify their decision if problems occurred.

Fasting of patients undergoing sedation for eye surgery is not necessary in most circumstances, although each department should have a standard protocol which is used with regard to this. It is particularly important in the elderly, children and diabetic patients to avoid prolonged periods in which there is reduced fluid intake.

Any sedative technique that is used should be reliable and controlled, with a smooth onset and recovery. Coughing or snoring can cause problems with raised intra-ocular pressure. It is probably best to utilise a technique for sedation that involves a single drug, which is given in increments over time. Due to the delay in onset of effects, it is best that sedation is commenced, and the effects noted, before surgery starts. Most patients who are undergoing sedation will be able to be treated like any other day-case surgery patient. However, consideration should be given on an individual basis as to whether an overnight stay might be necessary (e.g. due to social circumstances).

If sedation is unsuccessful, it may be better to postpone surgery and re-list the patient for a procedure under anaesthesia. Whether this is possible may depend upon the stage that surgery has reached. It is not considered safe to perform general anaesthesia on patients who are not properly prepared for it, nor is it desirable to perform deep sedation, due to the difficulty in distinguishing between this state and general anaesthesia. If verbal contact with the patient is lost, urgent action should be taken.

Sedation in this group of patients carries all the usual risks, but in the elderly it can also include increased restlessness, which may lead to abandonment of the procedure. In addition, it is common for patients undergoing eye surgery to develop an alarming bradycardia in response to pressure on the globe. This usually resolves if surgery is stopped for a short period, but it may require the administration of an anticholinergic drug, such as glycopyrrolate or atropine.

Eye surgery in general, and cataract surgery in particular, is a high-volume rapid-turnover specialty. However, this does not mean that the requirements for proper pre-operative assessment or peri-operative care should be relaxed. In some organisations, one anaesthetist can be allocated to two eye lists – one which contains high-risk patients, who may require 'hands-on' anaesthetic intervention (general anaesthesia, sedation or intensive monitoring), and a second list running simultaneously which contains low-risk patients undergoing straightforward surgery, in which the risk of requiring anaesthetic intervention is regarded as low. The anaesthetist would need to be familiar with both sets of patients, and the second theatre team would need to be aware that the anaesthetist could not leave patients anaesthetised or sedated in theatre 1 to attend to a problem in theatre 2. It is essential that such lists are properly organised, and that all members of the theatre team are aware of any changes or additions that have been made.

LEARNING POINTS

- Sedation is used to facilitate numerous treatments and procedures.
- A sedationist will need to be aware of the risks and complications that can occur in relation to particular procedures.
- It is best if sedationists are part of a team that provides a regular service to particular groups of patients undergoing specialist treatments.

References

1 Boodhoo L, Bordoli G, Mitchell AR *et al.* The safety and effectiveness of a nurse-led cardioversion service under sedation. *Heart.* 2004; **90:** 1443–6.

2 Whitaker D. Anaesthesia for cardioversion. In: Colvin JR, editor. *Raising the Standard. A compendium of audit recipes for continuous quality improvement in anaesthesia.* 2nd ed. London: Royal College of Anaesthetists; 2006; www.rcoa. ac.uk/docs/ARB-section6.pdf (accessed 14 August 2007).

3 National Confidential Enquiry into Patient Outcome and Death (NCEPOD). *Scoping Our Practice.* London: NCEPOD; 2004.

4 American Society of Anesthesiologists. *Statement on Granting Privileges to Non-Anesthesiologist Practitioners for Personally Administering Deep Sedation or Supervising Deep Sedation by Individuals Who Are Not Anesthesia Professionals;* www.asahq.org/publicationsAndServices/standards/39.pdf (accessed 2 August 2007).

5 American College of Gastroenterology. *Three Gastroenterology Specialty Groups Issue Joint Statement on Sedation in Endoscopy: a joint statement of a working group from the American College of Gastroenterology, the American Gastroenterology Association and the American Society for Gastrointestinal Endoscopy;* www.gi.org/physicians/nataffairs/trisociety.asp (accessed 3 August 2007).

6 Trummel J. Sedation for gastrointestinal endoscopy: the changing landscape. *Curr Opin Anaesthesiol.* 2007; **20:** 359–64.

7 Charlton JE, Jackson I. Endoscopy under sedation. In: Colvin JR, editor. *Raising the Standard. A compendium of audit recipes for continuous quality improvement in anaesthesia.* 2nd ed. London: Royal College of Anaesthetists; 2006; www.rcoa. ac.uk/docs/ARB-section6.pdf (accessed 14 August 2007).

8 Pearman T, Loper M, Trieryl L. Should psychiatrists administer anesthesia for ECT? *Am J Psychiatry.* 1990; **147:** 1553–6.

9 Pippard J. Audit of electroconvulsive treatment in two National Health Service regions. *Br J Psychiatry.* 1992; **160:** 621–38.

10 Bowley CJ. Anaesthesia for ECT. In: Colvin JR, editor. *Raising the Standard. A compendium of audit recipes for continuous quality improvement in anaesthesia.* 2nd ed. London: Royal College of Anaesthetists; 2006; www.rcoa.ac.uk/docs/ARB-section6.pdf (accessed 13 July 2007).

11 Royal College of Anaesthetists and Royal College of Ophthalmologists. *Local Anaesthesia for Intra-Ocular Surgery;* www.rcoa.ac.uk/docs/rcarcoguidelines.pdf (accessed 22 February 2007).

12 Rocha G, Turner C. Safety of cataract surgery under topical anaesthesia with oral sedation and without anaesthetic monitoring. *Can J Ophthalmol.* 2007; **42:** 288–94.

Index